FIT AND FIRM FOREVER

Your Personal Guide to

Losing Weight With
The Power Of Your Mind

FIT AND FIRM FOREVER

Your Personal Guide to
Losing Weight With
The Power Of Your Mind

Healthy Weight Control

By Motivating Master Hypnotherapist

M. Vance Romane

M.V.P. Ltd. Publishers

Canadian Cataloguing in Publication Data

Romane, M. Vance, 1949-

ISBN 1-894349-06-7

Printed in Canada

M.V.P. Ltd. Publishers
PO Box 75177, White Rock Postal Outlet, White Rock, BC Canada V4B 5L4
1-800-665-4656   (604) 538-1111   Fax: (604) 538-8477

Contents

Tips, What Is Holding You Back From Moving Your Body?, Additional Health And Fitness Tips, Smoking For Weight Loss, Loving Your Body, The Right Body Shape For You!, Read This To Motivate Yourself To Move That Body!

Chapter 1

Lose Weight Starting Today

The Foundation For Personal Weight Control

I have been helping people to lose weight for over three decades. During those many years, I have always found it most fascinating to research weight control programs. As I studied this field of knowledge, I constantly came across confusing contradictions. In this book, you will find practical techniques to help you lose weight, once and for all!

As one studies the field of obesity, it becomes apparent that, along with cigarette smoking, we have two of the most preventable causes of death. Each year 300,000 people in the United States alone die due to obesity conditions, and 400,000 due to cigarette smoking. My goal is to help you to control your weight, and at the same time to help you achieve a healthy body and mind, and to control your own emotions.

About the year 1900, one in twenty-four people developed some form of cancer. In the 1980's one in four people were diagnosed with cancer. In the 1990's, about one in three were being diagnosed with cancer. Just after the year 2000, it is predicted that one in two will be diagnosed with cancer at sometime in their life.

There are many different types of cancer, some of which have a much higher death rate than others. However, since our cells and all the chemicals in our body are made from what we eat, it is possible to have a lifestyle of healthy eating that will assist us to be healthier by boosting our immune system. Why not eat foods which keep you healthy and build a strong immune system as well as keep you lean?

In 1996, I was feeling very healthy. However a number of stressful situations entered my life simultaneously. I lost about eighteen pounds in a couple of weeks, which was a lot for me, as I was only about 5'6" and 150 pounds, before the weight loss. At the same time, although I had recently bought new glasses, I found I could not read the time on my video machine while sitting on my couch. Besides failing vision, I noticed my heart beating rapidly when I lay down to sleep. I was informed by my doctor that I had a hyperthyroid condition. Several tests were done at my local hospital, and then I was diagnosed with thyroid cancer.

Thyroid cancer affects more women than men, and it is proven to be one of the "safer" cancers. However, my physicians informed me that I had a very dangerously aggressive form of thyroid cancer. On Jan. 29, 1997, I had my entire thyroid gland removed. Meanwhile, numerous other stressful events continued to harass me. Believing in the "buckshot" approach to healing, I decided to go to San Diego for immunology treatment at the Livingston Foundation Medical Center. During my two weeks there, lab work was done to analyse my blood and other bodily fluids, and I received large doses of vitamin C, given intravenously. I watched videos and attended lectures to help me to understand cancer. In addition, their psychology department helps patients to understand and control stress, and their nutrition department helps patients to understand what they should and should not eat in order to boost their immune system. I had to learn how to give myself injections of B12, tumour necrosing factor, immune antigen and red purified antigen. However, to me the most fascinating part of the program was the nutrition and cooking department. We learned how to cook healthy foods to strengthen our immune system, to help make it difficult for cancer to gain a foothold.

After I left the Livingston Foundation Medical Center, I was told to continue the injections, the stress control techniques, the nutritional food plans and to continue to take the plant enzyme, Similase, and also Dophilis and Bifidus (Dophilis and Bifidus are now replaced by Enterogenic Concentrate). In addition, I was told to continue taking large doses of multi-vitamins and vitamin C. I was also advised by my doctor at the Livingston Foundation Medical Center to return to the Center once a year for a medical examination. It is important to note that this program was not two weeks of attendance, and then go home and forget about it. This program was meant to be a *lifestyle* change. Similarly, to control weight permanently and to enjoy a healthy life will require a lifestyle change.

Many people hope to lose weight by using some gimmicks temporarily, with the hope of losing weight permanently even when reverting back to their old ways. Weight control demands *taking responsibility* for our own health. It demands the inner strength and feeling that you realise there is no question that you have a *choice* to eat or not to eat certain foods. Long term weight loss requires a lifestyle change for permanent success. This lifestyle change must be based upon sensible eating and exercise, with occasional minor changes you can live with and enjoy for the rest of your life.

I once read about a doctor who researched 3,000 ways to lose weight and she found that only two methods work. You probably know what they are. They are less food (less calories) and more body movement (exercise). Many people will say "I hate exercise". However, they will delight in saying "I love moving my body". Therefore, one needs to find exercises or body movement that he or she will enjoy the rest of their life. Of course, interests may change over the years, but most any type of body movement will serve the purpose. Alright, we both agree that body movement and the right foods in the right amounts should bring weight loss, unless there is a physical complication for which medical consultation is necessary.

We know what to do, but can we do it? We say we want to be in control of our own weight, but are we willing to take responsibility to make our own good luck happen? Is there a magic button somewhere on a human being to force him or her to eat the right foods in the right amounts, and to force body movement?

I have found that the only way to assist people to develop a consistent and permanent lifestyle change is to strengthen motivation. What are the reasons you want a slimmer body? Why do you want to lose those love handles or that spare tire? Is it for better health? Is it to look more attractive to meet a standard that movies, television, and magazines proclaim to be the "best body shape"? We have seen too much anorexia and bulim-ia induced by such mass media hypnosis.

Do you want to lose weight to feel better or to have higher self-esteem? Is it to feel lighter on your feet or to fit clothes better? Perhaps you wish to lose weight to be a role model for your children. Many years ago, a woman came to me, and requested hypnosis for weight loss. Her reason to lose weight was inspired by her young daughter. Her daughter said "Mom, why can't you ride your bicycle beside me like all the other moms do with their children?" This woman said she was so embarrassed she did not know what to say to her daughter. She told me that the reason why she did not want to ride the bike was because she was embarrassed about the size of her thighs. In fact, she cried as she told me her story.

Now, do some soul searching and find out the strong, powerful, emo-tional reasons for you to be in control of your weight and fitness level. When you write down your reasons, write down and focus upon what you DO want, but never what you do not want. If you suggest an affir-mation to yourself to avoid something, you will be reminding yourself of the very problem you are trying to get rid of. Please take a few moments and write down what you want and the benefits you will achieve.

My reasons to lose weight - benefits for me!

_____

_____

_____

_____

_____

_____

_____

_____

Many people clearly know why they want to lose weight. They know the benefits of a more fit body, but, in spite of not having a physiological cause for the obesity, they still have trouble losing weight. They may use hypnosis, imagery, stress control, affirmations, self-esteem and assertiveness techniques, yet still have a hard time losing weight. This is likely due to the fact that the person has excessive stress or conflicts in their life that may only be dealt with by a trained psychologist or a very skilled counsellor. Counsellors have vastly different training. A good therapist or counsellor should only work with patients in their area of expertise. If you have used every method you can think of to control your weight, but have not been successful, I urge you to see a trained professional in the mental health field.

It is important to understand that having an emotional stress or conflict in your life and seeing a counsellor or psychologist is no different than seeing a doctor for the flu or a broken leg. In fact if this is needed for success, then the sooner it is done the better. Once serious stress and conflicts are reduced or completely removed, people usually regain a strong *feeling* of self-control, perhaps not known for many years.

I often advise my clients to write their positive reasons or benefits surrounding weight loss on a small wallet size card. I suggest that you do this and keep the card in your wallet. When you are in a bank line, a grocery line, waiting at the pump for your car's gas tank to be filled, sitting in a bus or air plane, or whenever you have a few seconds, read the benefits of having a healthier body and mind. Remember, like magic, we generally become what we focus upon.

It is stated by hypnotherapists that we have an outer conscious mind and an inner sub-conscious mind. In other words, although we may consciously want to do something, our motivation and lifestyle change will be far easier and more lasting if we place positive suggestions, affirmations, images and experiences into our subconscious mind before we fall asleep at night.

At one time or another, most people have suggested to themselves, just before sleep, to wake up at a certain time, and they do so, without an alarm clock. For many years, hypnotists, business people, Olympic champions, etc., have programmed their minds with positive affirmations and images just before sleep. The usefulness of this technique is unlimited, for we become what we think the most about. However, as the old saying goes, be very careful what you think about, positive or negative, for you will probably get it. For example, I believe that having a great fear for something such as a heart attack, cancer or even death itself may cause such an event to occur. Remember, "that which I hath feared has come upon me".

Chapter 2

It Starts At The Grocery Store!
Out Of Sight, Out Of Mind

Weight Control Is Different

Weight control is slightly different than controlling other habits like nail biting or smoking. You may cease biting your nails or stop smoking permanently and still live, but you cannot stop eating forever. Therefore, even though you may eat smaller quantities of food to stay alive, there is always the possibility that you may eat too much.

I will teach you the best types of suggestions to impress upon your conscious and subconscious mind during this weight control program. You will be steadily and consciously watching your habits in order to change them. This is not easy work. However, with hypnosis, it can often be remarkably easy.

Upon establishing a pattern, you will have to *work at maintaining your new habits.* Of course, it will be significantly easier once you have established better habits. Some authorities claim it takes from one to two years for the average person to completely reverse their habits and ways of thinking about food. This time for permanent change can be dramatically reduced with hypnosis.

Change Starts at the Grocery Store

Let's face it. The whole program must start at the market or grocery store. When I go shopping, I consciously try to avoid placing items in my shopping basket that are greasy, fatty or sweet. Occasionally I will "treat" myself to a chocolate bar or pecan pie, or something else that is loaded with calories, but this is rare, and seldom occurs during weight loss. However, after you have attained the weight you wish to be, a rare, but occasional "treat" may be permitted. Just before I go to the cashier in a supermarket, I usually look back into my shopping basket and search it, double-checking for "junk or garbage food". I will often take items back to the shelves, or just tell the cashier I've changed my mind on buying something.

If you live alone, it is easier to stock your shelves only with items that are healthy and nutritious. If you are able to convince others with whom you share a home to adopt new, healthy eating habits, your task will be easier, since each of you will be supporting and encouraging the other. If you cannot help others to change their eating patterns because of their lack of interest, there is no use creating tension-producing arguments. You will have to learn to eat the proper foods in spite of a lack of interest by other household members.

Habits are created by association and repetition. When I was young, we all bought a box of popcorn as soon as we entered a movie theatre. Now, I sometimes feel like having popcorn in order to enjoy a movie fully. Similarly, if you always eat in bed, while on the telephone, in front of the television, or at your desk, you are creating potential habit connections which may make you desire food whenever you recreate the situation. If you always eat while watching television, you may have developed a habit that creates hunger feelings, even though you may have already eaten. The eating-place should then become associated only with eating. This should be at the kitchen table.

When You Eat, Focus On Eating

It is important to be conscious of your food while you eat it. Nothing else should be happening while you eat, except perhaps a pleasant conversation. Even radio may become associated with eating. By enjoying the good taste of every single bite in a total way, by chewing the food thoroughly, you should feel satisfied with less food. Overweight folks usually gulp down food without proper chewing. This, as other bad habits, can be changed or unlearned. By chewing food slowly, and being in a relaxed state (i.e. not worrying about your personal or business life while eating), you will have greater salivation and it will be easier for your body to digest the food. Also, you will feel full with less food.

Eat Less And Be Trim

Make certain you have small quantities of food on your plate. Temptations will be reduced. At least in North America, most of us have been trained since early childhood to clean the plate or feel guilty. You can always get more food, but start off with a small quantity on your plate. It may be enough.

Another good tactic is to use small spoons and forks. This will make it easier for you to eat more slowly, and to chew your food more thoroughly. It seems like you have eaten more food if you use small utensils, and thus have to make more trips between the plate and your mouth. You will eat more slowly and feel full with less food.

Slim people often tell me that they are not very interested in food, that they have better things to do than to eat. They say: "I don't live to eat, I eat to live." You can develop this lack of interest or boredom towards food by externalising your interests, for example, exercise, walking, swimming, finishing old tasks, starting new ones, or generally having more important things to do. Make a reference list:

More important things for me to do than grazing are:

_____

_____

_____

_____

_____

_____

_____

_____

Three Meals a Day

Unless you have a medical condition that prevents this, you should try to develop the habit of eating three meals each day, at approximately the same times each day. These "sit down" meals need not be large, but you will be helped *to break the dangerous snacking habit.* If you continually eat at odd hours, your body will begin to feel hunger continually. Tell your self: "I eat three meals each day, *no matter how small.*"

Praise Yourself

Every time you resist a temptation to eat something you should not be eating, either at home alone, at a social gathering, or at work, be sure to stop for a few seconds and think of how proud you are of yourself. Develop a feeling of pride and accomplishment; the thought of success. Like an approving pat on the head to a good child, you will be rewarding yourself and slowly breaking and shattering old habits. Another way to reward yourself is to save up money in a small bank or a separate savings account that would have been spent on "junk food" in the past. When you have enough money, treat yourself to some small luxury such as a ring, a new watch, a week-end trip, or something that will give you happiness.

Those Last Few Pounds

During the latter part of your program, you will probably not notice too much weight loss. The last few pounds are the hardest to lose. BUT REMEMBER, *you must continue parts of your program* after you have reached your goal and your ideal weight. This continuing program is important for WEIGHT MAINTENANCE. Most people lose four to eight pounds per month. Again, slow weight loss is usually more permanent weight control. You create a more lasting lifestyle change over time.

Healthy Eating

You should become totally familiar with healthy nutritious foods. Your own physician or nutritionist will give you the best advice, and many good books are available in libraries, free of charge, to further expand your knowledge. One thing is certain. You can eat a lot of food and still lose weight, but it must be the right food, cooked properly. The sweet and greasy must be avoided. Avoid trimmings like sour cream, salad dressing and gravy. None should be used during weight loss. You may be able to use a little occasionally during weight maintenance.

When you are ready, you will lose weight

Chapter 3

Mind Over Mouth: The Power of Thought

The Power Of Imagination

Your will power comes and goes. Before my clients see me, they say will power mostly goes. Psychological experiments tell us that when the imagination and the will are in conflict, the imagination always wins. In Romane Hypnosis Seminars, we capitalise on this law to help people to change their feelings, attitudes and behaviour. Several examples will be given. Choose the ones that seem the most powerful to you.

On occasion, no doubt you have had dreams that seemed so real that it was hard to tell if you were dreaming or really experiencing what is happening. When you have deeply relaxed and concentrated your mind with hypnosis you should create dreams of ideal success, with your imagination. This is something like daydreaming, when your mind wanders. But in this case, you will set the track of the type and course, of the daydreams. They will not occur by chance, but you will become the writer and creator. You will present these daydreams to yourself during self-hypnosis, and just before you fall asleep at night.

Focus Your Mind For Success

First of all, you allow your body and mind to become relaxed. This will open the doors to the use of imagination and the acceptance of suggestion. What can the imagination do? Well, we seem to become what we think the most about. If we are able to present enough EMOTIONAL FEELING TYPE suggestions IN TERMS OF PICTURES, NOT JUST WORDS, we can eliminate bad habits and learn a new lifestyle that becomes a habit. You must take time to create the images that you feel will motivate you. To raise the voltage power of the suggestions, you can use all five senses of imagination and memories during the same sessions.

If you were on a "lucky streak", and everything you did seemed to turn out right, you would be building up a powerful form of self-confidence that would make it more likely for you to succeed in other ventures. I cannot build up this confidence in you very easily in real life, but I can in your imagination, and by the retrieval of success memories. This new feeling of power and control will transfer to your daily life and you will feel confidence to do just about anything new.

If we think about ourselves as being successful often enough and intensely enough, we are more likely to be successful. You see, the images you present to yourself with self-hypnosis and just before you fall asleep at night become accepted by your subconscious mind as *if you really had experienced success*. The subconscious mind cannot tell the difference between real and imagined success experiences.

When in a deeply relaxed state of mind and body, you may wish to imagine yourself already thin, as already having reached your goal. The mind affects the body. By thinking of yourself as having already reached your goal, your mind will start to alter your buying habits and your eating habits right at the grocery store. The mind is powerful. As an example, females will often experience symptoms of pregnancy without being pregnant, IF THEY REALLY BELIEVE that they are pregnant. Your mental, physical and emotional health, your relationships, your happiness, and every aspect of your world, is tremendously affected by your mood and thoughts.

Imagine Yourself As Thin

Think back to how you once looked or think ahead to how you will look. Imagine that the future is *now*. Imagine yourself cycling, or walking on a beach, with heads turning in admiration of you, or finding on a store display rack clothing that easily fits to your body. Imagine the exact size, shape and body contours you wish to have. Thin, trim, slim, fit, firm, slender and beautiful. Pause and think how you feel. So proud you are because you have already now attained your goal. Use all your five senses. What do you see, hear, smell, around you? What feelings do you sense on your skin, inside your body, and in your mind? Are you experiencing a particular taste?

Imagine Yourself At The Table, At Home, Work, Restaurant, At Social Gatherings

Imagine and see yourself putting a small portion of food on your plate; putting a small portion on your fork or spoon; eating very, very, very slowly; chewing thoroughly; the feeling of food entering your stomach; the experience of a slightly BLOATED feeling. Think that you feel SO FULL, with small amounts of food. Remember the full feelings you've had in the past. As the food enters your stomach, imagine it *expanding and bloating you*. Imagine you feel *so full with small amounts of food*. Think about how you are in better health, you have more energy, you are lengthening your life, you are enhancing your self-appreciation. Imagine yourself pushing away, refusing, turning down greasy, fatty, fattening and sweet foods at the table or social gatherings, and free sample foods in stores.

Imagine yourself shopping for healthy foods in grocery stores and the feeling of pride for refusing to buy unhealthy foods, and how happy you feel as you travel down the aisles putting only nutritious foods into your cart.

Picture yourself *leaving food on your plate and feeling glad about it*. Perhaps you give it to someone else, save it for another day, or throw it away. Concentrate on how it is even better for the food to go to waste than to be wasted on your waist.

In general, concentrate on the idea that your self-control is steadily increasing; that you will find it EASY and EFFORTLESS to do whatever you should and ought to do; that your desires to eat excess food or unhealthy foods are growing weaker and weaker, and that you will find it easy and effortless to eat sensibly; that your will to diet and eat the right foods in small amounts will increase every day; that you will develop a liking for healthy foods and a disgust, distaste, dislike or hate for "junk" food. Perhaps junk food should be illegal. The goal is to know that you are in control of what you eat or do not eat.

Imagine others around you gorging and greedily swallowing all the food that they can get, while you feel satisfied eating small amounts, eating slowly. Imagine wondering why they behave as they do. Wonder why they are unable to do what you can easily and effortlessly accomplish.

Eliminating Those "Tough" Foods

If you have particular food problems such as potato chips, soft drinks, donuts, butter, chocolate bars, pies, etc., specific imagery using association to disgusting thoughts may be helpful.   For example, imagine worms, a mouse, a rat, maggots, lice, urine, feces, snakes, cockroaches, human and animal hairs, etc., in a coke bottle as you open it. Imagine drinking it and vomiting all over the house or in a restaurant where everyone is staring at you.

Clear your mind with a visual image of blackness or white light surrounding you. Now imagine yourself refusing and turning down the same item, and you feel so good, so proud of yourself, in complete calm control.

Have you ever eaten a favourite food just before you felt nauseated with the flu? Likely you did not want to eat that food, or even look at or smell that food for some time after the incident. Thus, the favourite food and the ill feeling had become *associated*.

The more disgusting, the more real the purposely-paired association seems, the more you will be helped. You can use all the senses. Imagine the greasy feel of food as it goes into your body and how it slides around in your stomach. As you look at the food image in your mind, IMAGINE coatings of grease on it, bugs on it, etc. You must do this 1, 5, 10, 50, 100 maybe 200 times to benefit. The number of repetitions required depends upon the clarity and personal emotional voltage of the image.

In your Romane Training Program, a few clear image scenes are better than many less-defined images. If you do too much, you will dilute the benefits. Choose your goals, choose your images, make them clear, and real, and then repeat them. The more you think of your goals, both in and out of your concentrated relaxation sessions, the more you will be helped to reach that goal.

You Are The Boss Of Hunger

Another useful image to experiment with is what I call HUNGER CON-TROL. For example, if you are hungry, imagine yourself twice as hungry. Now imagine yourself as three times as hungry and so on until you feel you could clean out an entire health food store. Now decrease the hunger and go backwards until you imagine yourself as no longer hungry. In fact, imagine yourself as totally satisfied in terms of appetite. Then, imagine yourself as full, bloated. This exercise helps you to realise that if you can increase your hunger feelings, you can also decrease the same feelings. So have some imaginary fun creating total, zero hunger, and a bloated overstuffed feeling.

Repeat. Repeat. Repeat. If you are really serious about losing weight, you will practice what I have talked about as much as possible. Visualise at night before you fall asleep, in the morning, and before meals. It just takes a couple of minutes each time once you get the hang of it. For those who are less motivated to do this much work, in the evening before falling asleep is the best time for a once a day impression. Remember to get enough physical exercise and movement of your body parts to burn up the fuel you put into your body. Make sure it is high quality fuel and that you are not running on "garbage". You will experience better mental, emotional, and physical health. Before sleep, imagine yourself going out in the early morning for a brisk walk in the fresh air.

When You Eat The Wrong Foods Or Too Much Food

Fill in an alternative action response you will use to make the miseating mistake less likely to happen again, until it is extinguished for good.

Write down your trigger situations or feelings:

What Causes You to Eat too Much:	Alternative Actions Next Time:
Example: Anger	Go for a brisk walk
Eating at a Buffet	Avoid restaurant or eat from menu
	Be assertive - ask management for
	help with a specially prepared meal

Success Breeds Success

Write down your victories and read these before sleep to build your confidence:

Example: "Dec. 25, I received a box of very sweet chocolates and I gave them away."

_____

_____

_____

_____

_____

_____

_____

Powerful Help From Romane's Personal Notebook

- There are ONLY TWO WAYS TO LOSE WEIGHT: fewer calories (especially fat calories) and more exercise (body movement).

- Begin your day with exercise before breakfast and burn up the most calories with the least effort. Increase your metabolism.

- Eat a hearty breakfast selected from many food groups. It will give you energy for the day and you can burn if off throughout the day.

- Eat from all the food groups at lunch and dinner and feel full with less food. The more variety and colour on your plate, the more nutritious the meal. Eat organic food if possible.

- Regularly review a motivational card with YOUR PERSONAL REASONS TO BE LEAN AND TRIM. Write *positive* reasons to repeatedly read on your motivational card. For example do not write: "I don't want bad legs." Instead write what you do want: "I want strong, healthy legs."

Example: I want to be TRIM, FIT, FIRM, AND SEXY. My benefits are:

_____

_____

_____

_____

_____

- Drink two quarts of water daily, unless you have a medical problem preventing this as part of your program. I drink an entire glass of water every time I take my vitamin pills, or when I visit the bathroom. I drink more if it is a hot day.

- Read this book frequently for new ideas and reinforcement. Every reading will release new ideas, and further motivate you to do what you know you should do.

- Choose carefully what you think about, you will probably get it.

- Learn what foods are high, medium and low calorie. Get a small calorie book at your library and make notes or purchase a small calorie information booklet at your bookstore. Compare low calorie foods with the ones you used to eat.

- If your physician has prescribed a specific meal plan for you, this book will motivate you to follow it with enthusiasm.

- Eat mostly low and medium calorie foods from many different food groups for a balanced nutritious food management program.

- There are 3500 calories to the pound. Examples: one donut daily for a year adds sixteen pounds of fat; a small piece of apple pie with no ice-cream daily for a year adds forty-three pounds of fat. Little things do count.

- Develop a dislike for greasy, oily, fatty, and sweet foods.

- Be careful how you cook foods, avoiding grease, and high calorie oils. Steam, broil or bake your food. Sauté in water instead of oil.

- Occasional miseating is ok.

- Taste a little, know what the rest tastes like, and stop right there.

- Enjoy the natural taste of potatoes, bread, vegetables, salad, etc. without butter, gravy, sour cream, salad dressings, oils, etc. Use spices, and lemon juice.

- Do the work and you'll MAKE IT WORK!

- DECIDE AHEAD! "I'll be *more relaxed; full with less; I'm in control.*"

- "Your life is a direct mirror of the thoughts and experiences stored in your subconscious. Be careful. Control the door to the subconscious, your conscious mind."

- Dissolve false and phantom barriers to weight loss. Tear excuses apart. Be honest with yourself. Look after that marvellous body that is yours.

- Be ready for the ripples - or changes in other aspects of your life due to your adoption of new eating habits.

- Hunger may be interpreted as a good sign, the fat saying "good-bye".

> **Hunger is often only thirst. Drink water first.**

- If you really want dessert, have FRESH FRUIT, not canned. Avoid the sugary syrup.

- If you lose only one pound a week, that is over fifty pounds in a year.

- Alcohol has no nutritive value, but high calorie content.

- Nobody forces food into your mouth, you have control. You have even more control when you believe you do. Hypnosis helps you to believe you control you.

- Think trim, slim, lean, firm, fit, slender, shapely, sexy, great body.

- I omit adding sugar, salt, butter, syrup, jam, sour cream, gravy, salad dressings, chocolate bars, potato chips, french fries, and soft drinks when losing weight. If I do use them at all, I taste a little and know what the rest tastes like, and I stop right there.

- If you have children, teach them good eating habits. You want them to have easy access to jobs, dates, clothes, good health, and higher self-esteem.

- Leave some on the plate and lose weight.

- It is a sign of *self-respect* to treat your body and your mind well.

- Eat to live, not live to eat. DEVELOP OTHER INTERESTS; no need to fight it.

Will power strengthens with use. Set your weight goal. Be victorious!

Positive Attitudes And Pre-Planned Alternatives

- "Smiling is the most inexpensive make-up"

- "If you think you can, or if you think you can't, you are right."

- "Concentrate upon what you do want, not what you don't want. Forget "I can't because" excuses.... Focus on the detailed imagery and lifestyle changes for your certain success."

- "As in the past you fed your body too much or the wrong foods. Continue now to feed your mind new attitudes, new ideas, new skills, new experiences."

- "Be careful what you concentrate your thoughts upon... it will surely come."

- "Your current thoughts foretell your future."

- "You set your own limits by your thoughts and beliefs."

No More Boredom Eating

Here is what to do if you find yourself too bored to do anything but eat. Buy a pet; help someone in need; join a craft or hobby group; read a book; lie down and remember a favourite time; write a list of your good points; go for a brisk walk; have some fruit or juice; breathe deeply; listen to a relaxation tape; chew on cloves, a toothpick, a pen, a carrot stick, celery, gum; rub a coin, key or smooth stone in your hand; clean, floss, brush your teeth, use mouthwash; go to a theatre or library; relax in the sun; buy new clothing; phone someone you like; listen to your favourite music; plan a vacation day or holiday; tighten up your muscles and relax;

watch a favourite television show; watch a sunrise or sunset; buy a comedy record; have a shower and a shampoo scalp massage, a back massage; try something new; give someone else a back rub; use some hand lotion or new perfume/cologne; work in a garden; buy some flowers; buy yourself a present; go to a museum; take a child on a picnic or play a game of childhood again.

Chapter 4

How To Hypnotize Yourself

Choosing And Imaging Your Future - Finding Time!

Rapid, instantaneous self-hypnosis is available to those who believe. Instead of hoping for time to practice, you MAKE time. You deserve your time just as much as anyone else deserves your time! If not now, when? Before sleep; upon awakening; as a passenger; as a break during exercise, work, studying, as a "winding down" after work; or even in a library or a church. Powerful meditation helps weight control too. Auto-suggestion establishes the lifestyle change and repetition reinforces the permanence of the new you. Instant hypnosis can be done ten or twenty times a day, walking, standing or seated. "Sit-down" or "lie down" hypnosis is recommended one to four times a day. Begin with simple, easy to follow suggestions and work up to the more difficult ones.

Instant Self-Hypnosis

You can hypnotise yourself anywhere, anytime and give yourself quick suggestions. For example, if I am on a bus, or in a grocery line, I simply stare at a spot and place myself into a light trance and give myself a quick positive suggestion. The whole process can be as short as a few seconds.

Enjoying Hypnosis For A Better Life

Hypnosis is normal, natural and safe, something like daydreaming. You will never encounter any problems when you use self-hypnosis. However, never try to hypnotise anyone else, unless you have had professional hypnotism training. Problems are rare and only occur with inexperienced people hypnotising others.

Everyone experiences hypnosis differently. Reports sometimes include floating, tingling, heaviness, lightness, drifting, etc. Others feel that their consciousness has floated outside their body and they are looking at their body which appears limp, and totally relaxed. You will have your own unique experience which is yours alone, because everyone is a unique person.

The more you let go and just enjoy it, the more it will happen. You do not have to try hard to do anything. Just forget about everything for a while and R-E-L-A-X. You desire this time of quietness, rest and relaxation to focus your mind on health and success. All in life is achieved by concentration, in this case *effortless* concentration.

Misconceptions About Hypnosis

Here are some misconceptions many people believe. You might not awaken from hypnosis. People cannot keep secrets in hypnosis. You can be made to do anything in hypnosis. It must be perfectly quiet to hypnotise.

The *TRUTH* is that everyone comes out of hypnosis. People can refuse information and lie in hypnosis, if they want to do so. People CANNOT be forced to follow any suggestions that are of an illegal or immoral nature. And, I have hypnotised people in the middle of noisy exhibition midways, with thousands of people talking, shouting and applauding.

You do not have to make your mind "blank". Just relax yourself, and then seed the positive suggestions over and over and over into your mind. This will change your feelings, thoughts and behaviour, as you wish. After hypnosis, most people remember what has happened in the session. Some people forget a part of their session, however, it is hard to know if you forgot, if you forgot!

Simple Steps To Hypnotise Yourself

1. *Write out your suggestions positively*, what you want to accomplish. Pick a key one or two words which summarise the suggestion. Do not write what your do not want. Write what you do want.

2. *Hypnotize yourself.*

   a) Tense up all the muscles in your body and hold for 7 seconds. Then, relax and let go all over.

   b) Deep breaths. Breathe in through your nose and out through your mouth. Breathe deep into the bottom of your lungs. Lick your lips, letting your mouth open slightly with your jaw relaxed.

   c) Let your eyes roll upwards just a little, into your head, under your closed eyelids. Relax each part of your body. Drain away tensions.

   d) Think of a time and place when you were very relaxed. Use all your senses. For example, **see** yourself relaxing on the **warm, soft** sand of a beach; **hearing** the waves splash against the rocks; **feeling** the sand between your toes; **smelling** the fresh ocean air; **tasting** the ocean water. You can see, imagine or remember what it was like. When you remember a pleasant experience, you will **feel good**.

3. Think about the *one or two key words*. See, imagine your success as having been accomplished long ago. See yourself months or years in the future.

4. Think "at the count of five, I'll be wide awake, following all my suggestions automatically, effortlessly." Imagine yourself coming out of hypnosis feeling energised, healthy, motivated, and happy, or imagine yourself having a great restful sleep and awakening in the morning feeling refreshed, motivated, healthy and happy.

Creating Your Personal Auto-suggestions

- What is desired? What is the specific goal? What is proof of success for you?

- Be positive. Suggest what you want, not what you do not want. If you suggest what you do not want, you are reminding yourself of the very problem you want to erase.

- Summarise your suggestions in a few sentences and then into a few key words. Repetition of these key words makes them work.

- *Future projection.* See the successes as having happened long ago; that you have been successful for a long time already.

- Be patient. Some habits of many years may take days, weeks or months of suggestions of positive programming.

- Check with your own physician before giving yourself any medical suggestions. If you have a serious psychological or emotional problem, visit with a psychologist or psychiatrist privately.

- Many people do self-hypnosis on the bus, in their office, etc. for a relaxation break. At first, you might spend twenty to thirty minutes going into self-hypnosis. After a while, you will be able to go into it in a few seconds.

How Often Should I Use Hypnosis?

How often is hypnosis required to overcome a problem? This depends upon how strong your motivation is to overcome the problem, the type of problem, how long you have had the problem, etc. Just keep doing self-hypnosis as often as possible. Set aside one to four times daily to do self-hypnosis, and establish a habit schedule. Be patient for results and keep repeating positive suggestions on the areas you want to work on.

As you do self-hypnosis regularly, the everyday small irritations that used to upset you will lose their importance. You will be more relaxed and more in control of resisting stress.

Deepening Your Hypnosis Is Easy - Several Methods

"I'll go deeper and deeper relaxed......

- With every count from thirty to one."

- As I walk down each stair (in your imagination), go down the escalator, down each floor in the elevator, walk down the hill, etc."

- As I pump my index finger up and down."

- With every breath of air I breathe."

- Every second of silence that passes seems like an entire hour of actual relaxation in real world time." (Time distortion.)

- My right arm is attached to a pump. It is inflating with air. As it rises and touches my forehead, I go deeper. As it now falls, with every inch of floating back to my lap, I go deeper."

- I GO DEEPER WITH EVERY SESSION."

Chapter 5

Stress Management and More

Seven Secrets For A Happier Life

When you are happier, everything, including weight control, is easier and life is more fun. I would like to share with you some secrets for a happier life, in the hope of making your life even more satisfying.

1. **Pain Control.** There are many causes of pain. Check with your physician before using this technique. Sit or lie down comfortably. Close your eyes and relax. With your index finger of one hand actually draw a picture in mid-air of the pain. Draw the border or perimeter of the pain. Make the "drawing" as exact as possible. However, the "picture" should be done very slowly (about two minutes) and should be very large (about two and a half feet high/wide). This is usually excellent for headaches and many other pains as well.

2. **Snoring.** A common problem for families is one or more family members snoring. As ninety-five percent of snoring is done when the snorer lies on his back, sew a rubber ball into the back of the night garment or have a ball with a string tied through it attached to the sleeper.

3. **Positive Sleep Suggestions.** Experiments have shown that people can hear what is being said around them, when sleeping. One might whisper positive thoughts into the ear and mind of family members such as "When you grow up, you are going to be a very healthy, happy and successful person."

4. **Positive Pre-Sleep Suggestions.** You are very open to positive suggestions before sleep also. For example, people will often awaken at a set time they self-suggest before sleep. This is a good time to see yourself doing what you do want to do. For example, refusing fattening food, cigarettes, alcohol, gambling, etc.

5. **Before Surgery.** After having been given an anaesthetic, and just before you become unconscious, you are HIGHLY suggestible. In the movies of your mind, see yourself recovering rapidly, sleeping easily, having a good appetite, having been helped by a careful and skilled surgeon.. See yourself having prompt and regular bowel movements, prompt and regular urination. Incidentally, the mind still hears voices in the room, even under anaesthetic.

6. **Instant Relaxation.** Want to have a relaxation 'push button'? Get comfortable and close your eyes. Recall a time when you were truly relaxed: at a beach, in a canoe or sailboat, by a warm fireplace, in the woods, by a mountain stream, etc. Recreate the *sounds, feelings, sights, smells, tastes,* inside and outside your body. When you have reached a peak with the relaxation, rub the tip of the thumb and index finger of one hand together. Tell yourself as you press them together harder that you are intensifying the relaxation.

In the future, at a stressful time, or whenever you need to relax, just press the same index finger and thumb together. You'll be amazed how rapidly you relax.

7. **Instant Confidence.** You can also establish a 'magical push button' in the same way for confidence or optimum excellence. Just recall the times of your past when you felt that way. Recreate the scene with all your senses. The "button" could be the same two fingers of the other hand, a brushing of your leg, etc.

Some Possible Results Of Stress

- Headaches

- Stomach pains

- Depression

- Forgetfulness

- Insomnia

- Nightmares

- Sore neck or back

- Ulcers

- Hypertension

- Heart attack

- Fatigue

- "Burn-out"

- "Lump" in throat

- Temper

- Negative attitude

- Racing thoughts

- Digestive problems

- Susceptibility to illness

- Etc.

Listen to Your Body's Signals:
They shout at you to change your lifestyle.
Treat them like a red warning light.

Eliminate Stress And Gain Control Of Your Life:

- Talk to a friend, counsellor, minister or physician. **Follow your physician's advice.**

- Make an appointment for deep muscle massage. Ask your physician for a referral letter.

- Practice deep breathing.

- Tense up all parts of your body one at a time and let go and relax.

- Change your diet: less salt, less sugar, less alcohol, less fat, less meat, less coffee, be a non-smoker, drink plenty of water, eat lots of fruits and vegetables, and whole grain cereals.

- Listen to relaxing nature sound tapes, new age or classical music that induces slower, deeper breathing.

- Drive to a peaceful park, forest, beach, mountain or meadow.

- Exercise with a brisk walk, hike, swim, bicycle; go to a gym or buy/rent your own equipment.

- Play a stress reduction voice cassette or read a relaxing book.

- Take the day off or go on a vacation.

- Phone your local hospital to find out when the next stress reduction class will be given.

- Use self-hypnosis. Lie down and relax your body step-by-step. Remember a peaceful place in detail, using all your senses.

- Start a new hobby such as painting, ceramics, sailing, tennis, yoga, tai chi, etc.

- Be assertive, not aggressive. Take a self-assertion course at a school or university.

- Meditate: Sit quietly, eyes closed. Slowly focus over and over on one word, "calm" or "peace" or "relax".

- Have a warm bath at 92 degrees F. with pleasant bath oil.

- Drink camomile tea.

- See a foot reflexologist (foot massage) for better circulation.

- Listen to a comedy record; watch a live comedy show or video.

- Read a book on proper stretching exercises and do some everyday.

- Volunteer to help others for diversion, new activities, new friends. What will you have given during your lifetime?

- Change your daily routine, dress, route to work, furniture arrangements, etc.

- Set up a regular time to relax...a "relaxation break" instead of a coffee break.

- Change your attitude. Why does the same event bother some people, but not others? You have a choice. You don't always have to be right. Life is not always fair. Sometimes it's better to forget it than make it your mission to prove you are right.

- Don't be over-committed to do tasks. Find helpers to give you time to enjoy life. Work to live. Do not live to work.

- Avoid "keeping up with the Joneses". You may have everything you need to be happy right now.

- Make a daily "to do" list to tackle items in order of priority.

- Don't spend one hundred dollars worth of energy for a ten cent problem.

- Break down a major task into several small tasks. Remember the old story, you eat an elephant, one bite at a time.

- Set realistic goals. Is being the best or number one worth a heart attack or a lost relationship, if your time is monopolised by your work?

- Give compliments and enjoy taking compliments.

- Never say "I can't do this or that"...you get what you think about. Do not limit yourself.

- Make a list of tension reducers and things to do "to get outside yourself".

- Make your personal and family life a priority over other demands.

- Balance work with play, proper diet, sleep, exercise and relaxation.

Be thankful for your comfortable bed, friends, food, water, a chance to work, freedom and many other blessings.

> **Control stress – Gain mental and physical power and longevity.**

Chapter 6

Hypnotic Experiences and Mind Power

Were You In Hypnosis?

There are many indicators of developing and deepening concentration. You will experience some of these in varying combinations as well as in different degrees. Each time you enjoy hypnosis, you will experience a different altered state of consciousness.

Some Hypnosis Sensations:

- Arm, leg or general body heaviness.

- Floating, drifting, lightness.

- Watering of the eyes.

- Temporary numbness, tingling of hand, foot, arm, leg, etc.

- Time distortions: rapid passage of time.

- General body relaxation.

- Feeling good, comfortable.

- Small irritations no longer bother you.

- Lack of or little body movement.

- Sensitive hearing, attentive especially to the hypnotist's voice.

- Eyelid fluttering.

- Slowing of swallowing reflex.

- Slowing or loss of blink reflex.

- Facial features ironed out, soft facial expression.

- Pupils dilated.

- Feeling distant.

- Crystal clear memory of certain pleasant past experiences such as times of relaxation; when you had a strong will power, etc.

- Dissociation - a part of your body seems separated.

- Upward eye roll.

- Slowing respiration.

- Slowing pulse.

Relaxation Is A Major Key

It is a lot easier to say "no" to the wrong foods or too much food when you are relaxed. To accept the belief and realisation that hypnosis is successful for yourself, just do a before and after relaxation rating test. Zero can be total relaxation and ten can be extreme tension. Rate yourself before and after your session, and notice the benefits. Learn to be relaxed alone or with others.

> **Those who hurry to learn, learn little or nothing.**

The Power Of Your Own Mind

When I speak of mind power I refer to the power of imagery; the power of suggestion (hetero-suggestions) from a hypnotherapist, or auto-suggestions from yourself while in an altered state of consciousness; positive affirmations; relaxation training and any related techniques which help to reduce stress and give you a feeling of self-control over your life. Through thought power, I truly believe, one can cause self-inflicted death, or in many cases revival from the near dead, as in spontaneous healing. Our thoughts are now known to create thousands of chemicals that affect our feelings and emotions, and directly alter our behaviour. Our brain and body produce more different chemicals than a pharmacy. So, how a person thinks will drastically effect whether they are healthy or unhealthy. With every day that passes, I am more amazed at the power of thought and imagination. I will give you a number of examples to make this perfectly clear:

Tears

Tears of depression and sadness have different chemicals than tears of happiness and laughter. All tears look the same and feel the same, but they have different chemicals which are produced by our thoughts.

Lifting A Vehicle Off An Injured Person

Most people have heard of the story where an individual sees someone under a heavy fallen object. In shock the "helper" enters an altered state of consciousness and surprisingly is able to lift the object off the injured person. Is this story true? Yes, it is, and it has happened a number of times. However, the person doing the lifting usually ends up having injured their own body. Tests of muscle strength have been done with the same people hypnotised and not hypnotised. When they are hypnotised and told they are stronger, they show greater muscle strength than when they are not hypnotised.

Lemon Test

With a large audience, I will often demonstrate the lemon test. As I face the audience, I will speak about mind power for moment or so and say the following "...I have here in my left palm a fresh, juicy, bitter, bright yellow lemon. I am going to pick up this razor sharp knife with my right hand and slice this sour, bitter, juicy, yellow lemon in half. Oh! I almost cut myself! You should never cut something while it is in your hand." Then I place the knife down on the table with half the lemon. I take the other half and place the cut edge in my mouth. Then I make an audible noise as if I am sucking the sour bitter juice right into my mouth. Then I say, "How many of you noticed your saliva glands secreting saliva into your mouth as I talked about the lemon?" Almost everyone in the audience raises their hand. This is a dynamic example of the power of imagination instantly affecting our body.

I used to go to the grocery store for a fresh lemon for the demonstration. Now, I do the demonstration with an *imaginary* lemon and an *imaginary* knife. This saves me shopping trips and is easier to clean up, but the power of suggestion results are the same or greater.

Imaginary Perfume

Many years ago an instructor sprayed perfume in front of his students, and asked the students to raise their hand when they could smell the new scent in the air. Most students raised their hands. However, the bottle only contained water.

Digestive juices

Our body secretes different chemicals to digest different types of foods. In a research paper that I read many years ago, the hypnotised volunteers were told they were eating different types of foods. Interestingly, the same digestive chemicals were secreted in their body when they simply *imagined* eating certain foods. So, their mind and body interpreted the imagined food as real food. It would be possible to hypnotise some people who have certain food cravings and suggest to them that they have eaten those foods already, that they feel satisfied and full with the imaginary food.

The Voodoo Witch Doctor

I once read an article that claimed a Voodoo Witch Doctor had a success rate of healing equal to or better than psychiatrists. Of course Shamans often appear to have magical healing powers, and their function in their culture is of great importance. We have the often told story of the Voodoo Witch Doctor placing a curse of death on someone in the village because of some offence. This poor individual with the curse, whom we shall call

Mucumbo, has grown up witnessing the powers of the Witch Doctor. Mucumbo believes in the power of the Witch Doctor to cause certain death. Mucumbo becomes so obsessed with thoughts of his own death as being inevitable within days, such that he cannot sleep and he cannot eat. Perhaps Mucumbo begins to have hallucinations along with his delusions. Perhaps he becomes so distraught that he commits suicide, or perhaps he has a fear induced heart attack or becomes accident prone and falls off a cliff.

The Fraternity Student

There is a case of a young man who joined a fraternity. As part of his initiation, he was asked to lie on a table blindfolded. Foolishly, his fellow members shouted they were going to whack him on his throat with a knife. Simultaneously they whacked a towel across his neck. The new member died of a heart attack, literally frightened to death that a knife was about to slice his neck.

The Humanitarian On Death Row

Many years ago, I read of a case of a man in prison with a death sentence. A doctor approached this condemned man, and asked him to participate in an experiment to help medical science understand how the body works. This experiment involved the prisoner lying on a table with a small hole in his arm, so that the blood would slowly drain into a pail. The doctor explained that the experiment would determine how long it would take a person to die by such a method. The experiment began with the prisoner on the table, the pail, and the slowly dripping fluid. After a while, death was evident. However, the most interesting part of this experiment was that there was no hole in the man's arm and no dripping blood. What the prisoner heard was the dripping sound of water. Perhaps this self-fulfilling prophecy is again best explained by "that which I fear hath come upon me".

Cancer

I know of a case where the individual became so depressed he prayed for cancer, wishing to die. Within a short time he had cancer. After he got cancer, he asked God to remove the cancer. The cancer left his body. Prayer has power, but medical intervention is often necessary too.

Blushing

When an individual thinks a certain thought, he or she may blush. However, when a different individual thinks the same thought, he or she may not be embarrassed and does not blush.

Stage fright

When some people are asked to speak in front of a large group of people, their hands will tremble, their knees will shake, and their voice will quiver. Perhaps their heart will pound and their body will perspire, they may stammer and stutter, or their mind may go blank.

Another individual may come upon the stage looking forward to speaking to the audience, feeling relaxed, calm, and enthusiastic about sharing his or her thoughts with an audience considered to be friends, interested in what the speaker has to say. Not thinking of the audience as critical, the speaker also recognises it is impossible to please all the people all the time.

As a child, I used to be the most nervous public speaker. To overcome this fear, for about a month, each night just before sleep I imagined myself as a calm, relaxed speaker. This allowed me to feel calm speaking before audiences as large as 5,000 people, or to appear on radio or television shows broadcast to millions of people.

Self Imposed Limits

For many years it was thought that it was impossible to lift 600 pounds or run a mile in 4 minutes. After one person accomplished these feats, many others began to duplicate them. One hears the story of the baby elephant being tied with a rope to limit his movement to a small space. When the baby elephant grows up, it still believes it cannot break the rope. Then there is the story of fleas in a glass jar. With the lid on the jar, the fleas learn that they cannot jump out. Yet, when the cover is removed, they still cannot jump out as they have learned a shorter distance is all that can be reached.

Negative Identification

I believe a lot of people who expect and fear a certain illness, perhaps because a parent died of that illness, may induce the same illness by their thoughts. Similarly, I believe a lot of overweight people look at their obese relatives, and think to themselves, "I guess there is no hope for me, it is hereditary".

When someone labels the cause of their weight challenge as something unchangeable, due to heredity, or some other seemingly unchangeable reason, they may give up their power of self-control. They may fail to take responsibility to accept the fact that *only they can do what will bring the weight loss:* eat sensible portions of healthy food and exercise regularly. It is important to say to yourself, "I am a unique individual. There never has been and never will be anyone exactly like me. I am not my father, my mother, my brother or my sister. I am me, and I am one of a kind. I take responsibility for my present and future and I have the **POWER** - *the power of choice.* I am in control. I may be unable to change the past, but I can change my present, and my future."

Physiological Paralysis

In a case reported by Dr. W. J. Bryan Jr., a businessman signed a contract with a dishonest partner, and through his own written signature he lost a lot of money. His unconscious mind came up with a solution to prevent him from signing the wrong contract in the future. His writing hand became paralysed. This is the protective language of the body.

Tooth Extraction With No Local Anaesthetic

In my first book titled, *The Wellness Journey*, I gave a detailed account of how I hypnotized myself before the extraction of a tooth by my dentist. One of my techniques was to imagine numbness in my jaw that I had felt as a child, when the dentist would inject Novocain. By my recalling the sensations of the numbness, I believe I released natural chemicals that acted as a true anaesthetic. I not only felt no pain, but I did not even know when the tooth was extracted.

The Effect Of General Anaesthetic Nullified

When I was a young teenager, I was to undergo knee stapling in my right knee, under general anaesthetic induced by a needle to my right arm. As an experiment, I told myself in self-hypnosis that the needle solution was a bogus placebo and would have no effect. When the anaesthetic was injected in my arm, it had no effect and I remained wide awake and fully alert. Caution: Before using hypnosis in any medical or dental area, consult with your own physician or dentist first. They may have suggestions to assist you in the most effective wording of the hypnotic suggestions.

Pain Vanishes Instantly

As a young teenager I had a friend with a broken arm in a cast. I spent a couple of minutes hypnotising him, and about two or three minutes giving him hypnotic suggestions to remove the pain in his arm, that he said was so severe. When he came out of hypnosis, he said the pain was totally gone. Note: Hypnosis does not always work this fast for everyone, however, results are usually excellent if techniques are applied professionally. Some people need hypnotic conditioning or several sessions before hypnosis may have a strong permanent effect.

Instant Hypnosis

As a young teenager, I loved to do experiments with hypnosis. One day, I decided to go see my local pharmacist, Mr. Garnet. I asked him to give me an official looking prescription bottle with a label typed "Hypnotic

Pills". However, I asked him to put pills into the bottle that had no effect, and which were in effect placebos. The next day a friend of mine came over, and I asked him if he would like to experience hypnosis. He said "yes", and I told him that just one pill would rapidly induce hypnosis in him. He swallowed the pill and I couldn't believe my eyes. In about two seconds he began staggering, said he felt incredibly tired and immediately laid himself down on the couch. Seconds later, he had entered a very deep hypnotic state.

The Spirit Table

In my twenties, I had just finished reading a number of books by magicians exposing spiritualistic medium tricks. I was booked to present a lecture-demonstration in Cranberry Portage, Manitoba, Canada. I decided to try to do a demonstration called "table levitation". I asked for a table to be delivered to the stage. I expected a standard light weight banquet table. Instead, the volunteers brought a very large, rectangular table made of steel. This table was very heavy. I had doubts that the demonstration would work with a light table, let alone one so heavy. I did not want to ask for a lighter table, as I wanted the choice of the table to appear random.

Anyway, being one who enjoys experimentation, I asked for the volunteers to stand side by side around the table. I then asked everyone to place the palms of their hands flat on the table, and their little fingers touching the little fingers of the person next to them. I asked them to focus and concentrate on the thought of the table rising and lifting into the air. In a moment or so, this incredibly heavy table began to move several feet across the stage as though it was on wheels or had a mind of its own. The table also tilted, tipped, shook and rocked as though it were trying to rise. To say the least, I was astonished and I give you my word, I have never seen faces become more white more quickly than those of the volunteers, of which there were about 6 or 8. Believe me this table was heavy, *very* heavy.

So how does this work? It is known that our thoughts influence our body to produce unconscious movements. These are called ideomotor movements. What we think about is transmitted through the nerves to the muscles, and the muscles move unconsciously.

Pendulum Power

If you take a twelve-inch piece of thread, string, or fishing line and attach a fish weight, ring, or small crystal to one end, you will have a pendulum. Hold the end of the string about chest height with your index finger, and thumb of one hand. After steadying the pendulum to a stand still, relax the other arm at your side. Now, focus all your mind, your thoughts and your vision on the pendulum weight at the bottom of the string. There is no need for you to move your hand. Just forget about your hand. Now, focus on making the pendulum move in a circle, with your mind concentration alone. You may move your eyes in the same direction if that helps you focus. After you have been successful in the circle movement, you can make the pendulum move counter clock wise, left and right, and up and down. I have demonstrated this with hundreds of people and it works for most people. Again, the secret is in the unconscious movements by the hand holding the pendulum.

Mind Over Weight

Many years ago, Dr. Peter Lindner helped thousands of people, especially women, to lose weight. The technique that he advocated was self-suggestion before sleep. In a nutshell, patients were told to hypnotize themselves and imagine themselves as a lean, thin, slim person. This technique has proved successful over many years, and is still popular with many therapists as a tool to help their patients. The key is to use all your senses with imagination. That is, not only imagine yourself as if you were thin, but really be thin and imagine feeling that sliminess all over your body, *right now*. This helps to change what your eyes prefer to choose on a menu, where your legs take you in a grocery store, and what your hands prefer to choose to put in your mouth. I personally believe that with such mental imagery, whether you focus on the negative belief that obesity is your destiny, or on the positive belief that healthy and fit is your destiny, you can even change your metabolism.

Positive imagery of that slim new you will motivate you to move your body, and to eat sensible portions of healthy food. Again, as Earl Nightingale said, "We become what we think the most about."

Chapter 7

Getting The Drop On Moving: Lets Get Moving

How To Hypnotise Yourself To Lose Weight

1. *Atmosphere*: Darken the room, bring about quietness, unplug phone, etc.

2. *Get comfortable*: Loosen tight clothing, uncross your legs, do not have your hands on your chest. Preferably, lie down.

3. Stare at some light coming through a curtain or at a small spot that captures your attention or stare at a corner of the ceiling while lying down. Stare with your eyes only half open.

4. Inhale three DEEP breaths, in and out. Allow your eyes to close on the third deep breath.

5. Remember a time, a place when you were younger, *when you were very relaxed*, very, very, relaxed. Imagine hearing some of the noises of that place with your memory; *see* some of the people or things you saw; *feel* some of the things you felt; maybe even *touch* or *taste* some of the things you touched or tasted. Enjoy the nice memories all over again. You are preparing the field for the new plant.

6. Give yourself one to two weight loss suggestions at each relaxation session, the ones you have chosen or put together from the examples below.

Weight Loss Suggestions

1. You see yourself as THIN, SLIM, SLENDER, SHAPELY. See what it feels like to run, walk, swim, bicycle, ski, bowl, or? Hear the compliments of others, see the heads turning. It feels good. See your thin

face, slimmer calves, hips, small waist, smaller arms, etc. Feel, see your body EXACTLY as you want it. Hear yourself saying "no, thank you" as people you know offer you food which you simply are not interested in eating. You have other things on your mind. Enjoy the good feelings of seeing the new vibrant you in the mirror. Look how you're shocking old friends who have not seen you for a long time. Imagine looking at the thin you in the mirror and feeling each part of you - how slim. Imagine people calling you "SLIM" as a nickname. Make up similar suggestions that you like, daydreams that make you feel slender, healthy, good inside, and attractive outside.

2. Calm. Relaxed. "I now command myself to feel full, perhaps even a little 'bloated' with small and tiny pieces of food."

3. "I enjoy healthy and nutritious food, and feel full with small and reasonable portions."

4. "I dislike greasy, fatty, fattening and sweet foods. I have a definite dislike, distaste and disgust for such garbage food."

5. "I now *prefer* to LEAVE FOOD ON MY PLATE, to throw it away, or give it away; or store it for another day, INSTEAD OF putting it on my waist, where it would really be WASTED and just stored as unwanted fat."

6. "I eat and relax by chewing my food slowly."

> **A calm relaxed mind can do whatever it wants to do.**

Failure Or Success Created By The Imagination

Many years ago theatrical hypnotists would use this story to illustrate the power of the imagination. Imagine a very thick sturdy plank on the floor, ten feet long and one foot wide. Imagine walking back and forth across the plank as though you were walking on the floor or the earth itself.

Soon you will realise that there is no chance of falling off the plank. Now, let us take this plank and place it between two tall buildings. The plank will not bend and there is no wind, but the fall to the ground is 100 feet. Now, will you walk across the plank? Obviously very few would attempt to walk the plank unless this was done regularly as part of one's occupation. Chances are that the average individual attempting to walk the plank in mid-air would fill his mind with mental pictures of falling, slipping, dropping through the air, and a pile of broken bones lying on the ground. This fear and nervousness is more likely than not to distract the walker to such an extent that he would fall off the same plank he had walked upon time and time again.

The Power Of Hypnosis

I help thousands of people to stop smoking, lose weight, relieve stress, and build self-esteem. It is most amazing when someone stops smoking at the seminar and says: "I don't even remember why I came to this seminar". Another individual told us that after the seminar he not only became a non-smoker, but for some unknown wonderful reason he felt the urge to throw away all his narcotics.

Nature's Built In Alarm

I often ask my audience members if any of them sometimes go to sleep at night, and just before sleep they suggest to themselves that they wake up at a certain time, and they do, almost to the exact minute. Have you ever programmed your mind before sleep to awaken at a set time, and you did?

Uses Of Hypnotic Mind Power

Hypnosis today is accepted worldwide by physicians, psychologists, psychiatrists, dentists, social workers, ministers, the police, and many others as a scientific tool to help people to function with a healthier mind, body and spirit. The uses are unlimited and would be far too long to detail here. For more information please see my first book *"The Wellness Journey"*.

Body Movement:

I am writing this book in Kapoho on the Big Island of Hawaii. Everyday just before lunch, I go out snorkeling, to swim with turtles and colourful fish. As I swim, my stress melts away. I receive total body exercise and come out of the water feeling refreshed. Sometimes, while swimming, I even think about problems or projects I have to deal with. Physical activity makes me feel better and look better. It allows me to have fun while improving my health and burning up calories to control my weight.

On the other hand, there have been many times in my life where I have participated in different forms of physical activity, and then I lost interest in that activity. I have seen some people lose interest in an activity, and then stop moving their body altogether; assuming that they no longer like exercise. However, there are hundreds of activities one may choose from for physical activity. So it is important for you to have some choices. All you need is some types of body movement that you enjoy.

As someone once said to me, "if something is not working, try something else". This sounds obvious, but it is amazing how often people keep banging their head against the same wall. If one lives alone, he or she may wish to find a friend or neighbour, a partner to schedule a regular time, several times a week, for body movement. This appointment for yourself should be put on your calendar, as it is just as important as your appointment with your doctor or dentist.

If you live in a family, try to set a regular time several times a week with other family members for exercise. There are many activities that people can do that cost little or no money. If you are buying gifts for someone, or if someone wants to know what to buy for you, how about choosing a fitness gift from a sports and recreation store. Perhaps a professional skipping rope or a pedometer that measures distance walked and calories expended.

Here Are Some More Tips

1. Restrict sedentary time on the computer or watching television.

2. Instead of celebrating with your family or friends by going out for a meal, why not have everyone participate in an activity that has lots of body movement, and burns up calories.

3. Have a pet that you can take for long walks. You will be forced to take the dog out regularly.

4. It is not important to make these activities competitive, but rather emphasise the health and fitness aspect. Health and fitness should be given greatest importance.

5. Be sure to have a water bottle near by, to replace water lost during your physical activity. We are generally told to drink at least 8 glasses of water per day to stay hydrated. This would be more or less depending on the climate where we live.

6. During a work day, stop and stretch, or take a short walk a few times each day. This will keep you more alert and make you more productive.

7. Whenever possible, use the stairs instead of an escalator or elevator.

8. When you park your car, park further away for the exercise and fresh air.

9. Join a fitness group or gym with one or two friends so you will be more inclined to go consistently. An owner of a fitness gym once told me that he sells "tons" of memberships in early January, as people make their New Year's resolutions. He also said, "By the end of February hardly any of these folks are attending regularly." If not used, these memberships are not only expensive in terms of money,

but more importantly, in lost health. Secondly, you do not want that guilty or depressed feeling that comes from not completing your project, which is a lifestyle of fitness, *for life*. It is alright to occasionally forget fitness, especially if you are feeling ill, and your body needs all available energies to heal itself. Do not exercise before sleep, or you will end up with another problem - insomnia. So, if you want to succeed, make a plan. With no plan, all you can have is failure.

10. Instead of driving to places close to you, walk or jog there. Do not run on a hard surface like a sidewalk or road, or as my doctor says, "You'll end up with knee problems when you are older."

11 If you take a bus, or someone gives you a ride somewhere, you could ask them to drop you off a short distance away from where you are going for more body movement.

12. Enjoy chores such as cutting the grass, raking leaves, gardening, washing and waxing your car, shovelling snow, or house work. This will give you fresh air and body movement. I recently spent several hours digging weeds out of my garden with a shovel and with my hands. I have a nice garden and I enjoy working with the earth. I felt like a kid playing in the mud. It was fun!

13. Sometimes when I feel a little stressed out, I walk down to the beach and listen to the ocean waves. The small hills in White Rock, British Columbia, where I live, give me the gift of even better body movement.

14. When I am travelling on my tours, I enjoy seeing the local sights on foot. Maybe you like bicycling, canoeing, kayaking, water walking, nature hiking, golfing on a course or driving range, kite flying, catching a ball, playing softball, tennis, or racket ball, bowling, dancing, or participating in martial arts classes. Some people complain of the cold of winter, and others use it for their enjoyment such as: ice skating, tobogganing, cross-country skiing, or down hill skiing. It's best if you have a choice of several activities that you can pick to enjoy in all kinds of weather.

15. Visit your local recreation centre. Mine has a great gym for use at a very low cost, pay as you go membership. Many recreation centres have indoor and outdoor areas where you can play tennis, racket ball, volleyball, badminton, swim, etc.

16. I knew one wealthy individual who used to walk all over the city with a garbage bag, and he picked up litter, because he had great pride in the cleanliness of his city. He would wear light gloves and carry a stick with a nail on the end.

17. If you are like me and you are not excited about cold weather exercise, then if possible, walk in indoor facilities such as: shopping malls, jogging tracks, or large airports. These are often available in schools and colleges as well. You may contact the manager of a shopping mall, and suggest that you would like to organise a regular mall walk, and he may help you by advertising to spread the word. If your social life is lacking, participation in life through various fitness programs will help you make new friendships with people with compatible interests. In addition, walking up and down stairs can be quite a work out.

For personal interest, I used to interview people obsessed with exercise. Frequently, I was told that they would not even talk to people, let alone go out with them unless they were physically fit. I was quite surprised how strongly they felt about people not interested in exercise. One fitness enthusiast actually told me that he was disgusted with people who would not look after the marvellous body they were given. Developing friendships with people interested in fitness will motivate you to be consistent with your exercise program.

18. I once owned a home gym with about 7 pieces of equipment. The variety of equipment allowed cross training, and eliminated boredom by allowing for diversity by using different equipment on different days. My goal was not to build up muscle but instead to have better health and fitness, to increase my energy, to melt stress and even to improve my posture. Of course, regular exercise is a part of the life of most successful people. With better physical fitness the result is better mental fitness.

19. Be sure to go to the library or book store and get a good book on stretching, as this is very important before and after exercise. Your doctor or chiropractor will also provide you with information on stretching.

20. The new approach to weight loss and fitness is to think of exercise as absolutely anything that gets your body moving. It is important to keep in mind that any body movement burns calories and if one does not increase their calorie intake they will lose weight. So, there is no need to think that strenuous exercise is necessary, but, just keep moving those large muscles in your arms and legs.

21. For variety, many people are also using low impact aerobics videos at home. You might also purchase a video on stretching. Other good videos would be on breathing, yoga and Tai Chi. If you are unable to locate these locally at stores or libraries, feel free to contact us. I have even seen exercise videos advertised with nude instructors purporting to show body movements with greater clarity. According to the advertisers, these videos are guaranteed to maintain your interest and motivate you to exercise!

22. If you don't feel like exercise, just think about *how good you feel* after exercise. Think about the importance of a healthy heart and keeping your weight down. Hopefully you will be motivated to do something to bring back those good feelings again. After you have exercised consistently for a period of time, it will become a habit you will not want to miss, because you started off with a variety of activities that you really enjoy.

23. You can set a fitness goal such as when you reach a certain weight you will treat yourself to a massage, vacation, new clothing, etc. Be gentle on yourself. If you miss exercise for a short time, just remember how good you felt when you were exercising and get yourself back into the fun of body movements that you enjoy.

24. In the summer, go with some of your friends and visit farms, prefer-

ably organic farms. Pick yourself some fresh fruit such as strawberries, blueberries, apples, oranges, etc.

25. Many people like to keep an exercise log or calendar which lists the
day, type of body movement, duration, intensity (i.e. number of repetitions), who it was done with and how you felt (during and after).
Some keep this in a diary book. This diary book can help keep you
motivated when you read about the good feelings you felt after the
exercise, time and time again. Remember, the old idea of "no pain, no
gain" is no longer an acceptable idea. If you are feeling pain, that part
of your body needs a rest.

> **CAUTION:** Do not start any exercise program without discussing it first
> with your own doctor. If new to this, you will have to begin with easy
> exercise such as walking short distances, and then *slowly* increase your
> activity over time towards more strenuous body movement.

26. Many times people will begin an exercise program and push themselves to the limit. They become sore and exhausted and quit. Start
slowly and be patient and develop a new lifestyle. Learning a new
lifestyle for permanent results takes time.

What Is Holding You Back From Moving Your Body?

Everyone agrees that exercise is good for us, that it prevents obesity and
other diseases as well. Yet, talk is often not matched by action. People
will say that they believe exercise is needed, but they often do not do it.
Many people will say, "I am too busy; I don't have the time". I believe
that we often over stress ourselves with too much work and not enough
play. Many people spend much of their time working for extra money to
buy things they want, but don't need. Many people spend too much
inactive time on the computer, computer games, and television or hide in
books.

Many jobs today involve little physical activity, and instead we sit at a
desk for many hours. Instead of a coffee or snack break, perhaps it

should be a brisk walk break for some fresh air. We hear many people say physical exercise should be a minimum of thirty minutes per day, three days a week. I think it should be more. I also suggest that a firm appointment should be made on our calendar for exercise to be done at the same time each day. A better goal might be a minimum of 30 minutes of activity every day for better circulation, burning of calories, stress reduction, better health, etc. Even short periods of exercise such as ten minutes, where you are moving the large muscles of your arms and legs, as in brisk walking, can add years to your life and life to your years. It all adds up to present and future benefits. The danger is a sedentary lifestyle.

Corporations should set aside an in-house fitness room for employees, with showers. They should promote recreation activities, and games; promote walking groups; sponsor fitness seminars; make fitness literature available or perhaps even give complementary health club memberships to their employees. With healthier and happier employees, their business is more likely to prosper and there will be fewer days where the employees call in sick.

Additional Health And Fitness Tips

1. When you go to a restaurant, make sure it is one that offers low fat choices. Phone ahead to find out if they will accommodate you on the types of food that you choose that will be nutritious and tasty. Assert yourself! Ask for a personalised meal cooked to your specifications.

2. Do not attend buffets while losing weight. Instead, order from the menu. Do not go back for seconds.

3. Read the nutrition labels carefully. Avoid high calorie items and high fat items, or at least make the ingestion of them minimal.

Smoking For Weight Loss

An enormous number of people, especially women will smoke cigarettes in order to control weight. It is true that smoking does help to control weight for many people. When people stop smoking, one third *gain* weight, one third *stay the same* and one third *lose* weight. So the metabolism is effected differently in different people. However, I heard one doctor say that you would have to gain over 70 pounds of excess weight to equal the damage done to the body by just a one pack a day smoking habit. Of course two or more packs per day is much worse.

The answer from doctors is that it is better to quit smoking first and then work on the weight later, unless the patient is dangerously (morbidly) obese. If you need to stop smoking, contact me for my stop smoking program which combines stress control, relaxation training, self-esteem building, hypnosis and practically every other best stop smoking idea available. If you have this problem, I believe I can help you, as I have been helping people to stop smoking for over 35 years. Call 1-800-665-4656 or visit my web site at http://www.vanceromane.com

This year, over four hundred thousand people in America will die from smoking and over three hundred thousand people will die from being overweight. Obesity effects over one third of the adult population, and is becoming a greater problem each year world wide. Obesity in children is steadily on the rise as well, with a forty-two percent increase in child obesity since 1980. This is largely due to less exercise and more television viewing. *As I mentioned earlier there are only two ways to lose weight; proper nutrition with sensible portions, and exercise through body movement.*

It is also important for those who are working on losing weight to come to terms with conflicts in their life, as these can act as deadly road blocks to prevent success in all areas of their life. Thus, methods of coping with stress, self-esteem and even assertiveness are good for not only weight control, but also for success and self-control in life. If you need a therapist, take 2 to 3 sessions with several to see which therapist is the best for you.

Loving Your Body

Over the years I have found that we will lose weight faster if we love our-selves, including our body shape that we currently have. In other words, it is much easier to love the weight off than to hate it off. While the media of Hollywood movies, television, magazines and novels continue to pro-claim that slim is better in terms of sexual attractiveness, romance, and beauty, the dislike of our own body continues to grow. Stereotypes of the obese person not having self-control, being lazy or a lesser person con-tinue to abound with the inappropriate direct and indirect jokes on the street, and via the media including television comedies and comedians. Some non-medical results of obesity are: difficulty finding employment, no dates, loneliness, a lack of energy, low self-esteem, difficulty fitting into clothes, etc. Such stress can lead to infinite assorted medical and psychological illnesses, including suicide.

The media's responses of society towards people having the *disease* of obesity may create depression in the obese person due to their failure to lose weight, because of an unrealistic goal. Many people hope to be as thin as they were when they were young, or as thin as a friend or as thin as their favorite movie star. However, we are not all built to look the same and what a boring world it would be if we all did. It is most impor-tant that the person wanting to lose weight have a great love for them-selves and it also helps if they have a great gusto for life.

Some people are naturally larger boned though heredity, and others are smaller. Some people are tall in some countries, and others are short in other countries. In some countries, usually where food is scarce, obesity is looked upon as being desirable.

In some countries people mutilate their bodies and think it is beautiful, and obviously this has come to North America. In some countries people have stretched their necks, widened their mouths, bound their feet to make them smaller, and so on. So, what is the right body shape? I think the right body shape is the one that you have, or are about to have, which is the one where you are the most healthy and the most fit.

The Right Body Shape For You!

Remember, the goals you set for yourself should be short term and small. As you reach each of these goals, you will establish the "mind set" that you are a successful person. Small successes lead to greater successes. Your new life will be created one piece at a time. Too high a goal at once can seem overwhelming, and may lead to frustration and failure. So realistic goals and good self-esteem will make it easier to establish healthy eating and exercise habits. Redirecting all that time and energy that you used to spend on disapproval of your body to a new energy outlet will help you change your lifestyle. Keep studying: low fat, low calories, and this book. Keep moving your body, and learn new ways of meal preparation. This will bring you success.

It is not appearance we need to be concerned with as much as *health and fitness.* Twenty-two percent of children ages six to seventeen years old are now severely overweight, while thirty-three percent of the adult population is considered to be obese. We need to be concerned about preventing disease and premature death, which occurs too frequently due to obesity. Being overweight and inactivity are directly related to five of the ten major causes of death in North America, including heart disease, atherosclerosis, stroke, diabetes, and some forms of cancer. Obesity is also associated with many other medical problems including osteo-arthritis and gout. In terms of mental health, many obese patients suffer from low self-esteem, a sense of failure, hopelessness, depression and even suicide.

When parents share joy and excitement about participating in body movement for fitness and health, and schools, churches, community clubs, corporations and governments work together for the enthusiastic support of exercise, health and fitness, then many illnesses will vanish. When obesity is respected as a *disease* to be treated and helped like other physical illnesses such as a broken limb, then public awareness and support for treatment will function at a higher level. As an example of hindrance to promoting fitness and health, my brother attempted to set up an in-house gym and fitness centre in his place of business for his employees. Yet he was unable to do so due to government zoning ordinances. All he wanted to install was a number of pieces of exercise equipment and a shower, in his own building. He was denied this benefit for his employees.

Read This To Motivate Yourself To Move That Body!

1. Less likely to have a stoke, hypertension, cardiovascular disease, diabetes, breast and colon cancer, gallstones, osteo-arthritis, gout etc.

2. Less money and time spent on sick days at work due to illness and less time spent in the physician's office or hospital.

3. Less money spent on medications.

4. *Reduced* stress, anxiety and depression.

5. Better sleep.

6. Better concentration, clearer and more creative thinking.

7. Improved strength, endurance, and flexibility.

8. Improved appearance.

9. A feeling of control over your life and higher self-esteem.

10. Chances to meet new friends.

11. Improved bone density, with less chance of osteoporosis and fractures as you grow older.

12. Your improved health will bring you greater happiness in *all* areas of your life.

13. Build muscle tissue.

14. Prevent back problems.

15. Tone muscles.

16. Better posture.

Add your own reasons to move your body:

17. _____

18. _____

19. _____

20. _____

21. _____

Chapter 8

Eat Healthy And
Build Your Immune System Too!

When I was a cancer patient at the Livingston Foundation Medical Center in San Diego, I learned I had to strengthen my immune system. Let me share what I learned at the Livingston Foundation Medical Center to assist you to strengthen your immune system.

In order to strengthen your immune system, it is recommended some foods should be omitted, or limited in your diet. You should avoid chicken as it is contaminated with the potential to develop cancer. Commercial beef, and turkey also should be restricted or eliminated from the diet. Sheep, lamb, and wild game, however, are considered to be safe, or cleaner meats. Fish that have fins and tails are safe to eat, but not shellfish or other "scavenger" fish, as they store more toxins. However, because our oceans are becoming more and more polluted you should be careful and know where your food comes from.

A strict vegetarian diet is *recommended*. If you do not follow a strict vegetarian diet, then you should try to eat only the "cleaner" meats. The only eggs I would recommend would be the eggs you can purchase from the Livingston Foundation Medical Center. These eggs have been inoculated. They can be purchased six dozen at a time and UPS will deliver them. Eggs in the diet are optional, but they are a good source of protein.

Dairy

Butter and cream are acceptable, however, only in small amounts because of the concentrated fat. During weight loss I would not recommend them at all. Concentrated saturated fats may cause heart disease. Milk is not recommended. Too much fat can lead to colon cancer, so make sure you use it sparingly. The Livingston Foundation Medical Center recommends that if using cream, you use *heavy* cream, not half and half, and dilute it fifty percent or more with water. To do a large batch, you would mix one part cream to ten parts water.   However, it is recommended that you have no more than one pint of cream per week. Seed milk, soy milk, and rice milk all make a good substitute for milk.   If you don't like rice or soy milk produced by one company, try another company's version. They can taste very different. Tofu or tofu-soy cheese are recommended instead of cheese. Also, you can use nut and seed cheese for a different taste.

Sugars

The use of sugars should also be reduced or omitted from your diet. Sugars are found in cookies, cakes, ice cream, many commercial dressings, ketchup, pickles, etc.   It is recommended that you read the food labels to find out the ingredients. You will discover that the ingredients are listed in descending order, so if sugar is one of the first few listed, that food should perhaps be omitted or restricted from your diet. To be sure of how much sugar you are getting, it is best to make your own baked goods and sauces, so you can control the amount of sugar in these items. Also, avoid artificial sugars. They are not good for you, and may even cause cancer.

Foods that may be used in small amounts are:

- Butter

- Cream

- All oils

- Sugars. Sugars should only be used in very small amounts as sugar fuels cancer like gasoline.

- Clean meats and fish are acceptable in small amounts

> **Make changes slowly and after a while only the healthiest foods will taste good to you.**

Foods that may be used in moderate amounts are:

- Fresh fruits. Fruits should however, be limited to three pieces per day as they are high in sugar.

- Nuts and seeds.

- Soy products. Tofu and soy cheese contains fat so should only be used moderately.

Foods that may be used in larger amounts are:

- Vegetables that are juiced, raw, in salads, cooked, baked, or steamed.

- Whole grains (fibre), oatmeal, cereals, pastas and bread. It is recommended that you eat a variety, and not the same ones everyday. White flour products are NOT recommended.

- Beans and legumes. These are the "meat" of the diet. Beans are very high in protein.

Juicing

It is recommended that you drink one pint, or two cups of carrot juice per day. Other wonderful juices can be created with your juicer, such as a vegetable medley. Use a variety of vegetables with a variety of colours. Greens, beets and celery have beta carotene. Broccoli and cabbage may taste bitter, and should perhaps be used in small amounts. I would recommend a Champion Juicer, as I find it works perfectly for me. All juices, especially carrot juice should be ingested within twenty minutes to avoid oxidation. So you will need to make a fresh batch each time.

It is recommended that you make the staples in your diet high in fibre. Also, be sure to use a variety of vegetables, whole grains, fruits, nuts, beans and legumes. Fibre traps toxins and takes them out of the body. There are two types of fibre, water soluble, and water insoluble, therefore it is important to have a variety (balance) of foods. When increasing fibre to avoid constipation, increase your fluid intake.

Ultra Dophilus and Bifidus Dairy Free

These are friendly floras and are considered to be "friendly bacteria". They are very good for digestion and they inhibit "bad" organisms. Gas may increase as you go from a meat diet to a vegetarian diet due to indigestible carbohydrates, especially in the bean and vegetable group. You will have less gas if you take ultra dophilus and bifidus *one half hour* before you eat, especially if you are eating beans or vegetables. If you do not mix fruit with vegetables and beans, you will also produce less gas.

Water-soluble fibres

These are oats, oat bran, pectin, beans, sea weed, etc. When you eat these foods you will need to *drink lots of water.* Flax seeds are very good for you, but should be ground, as the whole seed is not digestible.

Oils

Some oils do not tolerate high heat. It is recommended that you avoid commercial processed oils, and use cold pressed oil instead. Easily available cold pressed, extra virgin olive oil is the best to use, but should only be used sparingly. When I was in Hawaii, I found an oil even healthier than olive oil. It is macadamia nut oil. If you are in Hawaii, you may wish to purchase a few bottles. Do not use the oil to fry, but instead use for sautéeing, as the oil is best when used at a lower heat. To consume less calories, sauté in water. Flax oil makes the cells of your body stronger and is also a very good oil to use. However, remember you should limit your intake of fats and oils to one to two teaspoons per day, or omit it completely. For example, when I go to a restaurant I use no more than one pat of butter, if I use it at all. For many years I dropped butter completely from my meals, and I never missed it at all.

Chapter 9

Healthy foods and a healthy lifestyle

You can build a strong immune system with healthy nutritious foods. This will give you a new lifestyle of healthier eating habits and a slimmer you. Nutrients are lost in foods due to pesticides and chemicals, time of long-distance transportation, warehouse storage, and over-cooking of foods such as boiling the nutrients out of vegetables.

Things that you should constantly remind yourself to be healthy, are:

- Avoid stress

- Avoid tobacco and alcohol.

- Avoid refined flour.

- Avoid white sugar.

- Avoid junk foods without vitamins and minerals.

- Avoid chicken, as all chicken seems to be infected with a cancer-causing organism called the PC microbe, according to Dr. Virginia Livingston.

- Avoid meats, due to pesticides in the animals, steroids that the animals are given to enhance growth, and the processing of sick animals. Many animals have disease and tumours inside their body and this is not detected by outside inspection. Cleaner meats such as lamb, wild game and fish may be eaten in small amounts as they have lower PC microbe, which is believed to be cancer causing.

- The key to a healthy diet is balance and variety, for a healthy mind and body.

- Missing nutrients can lead to a diverse assortment of conditions and diseases.

- Foods with high fat should be avoided.

- Lots of carbohydrates should be eaten, as they provide the most available energy to the body.

- Eat a variety of foods and maintain a balanced vegetarian diet.

- Eat *organically grown*, pesticide free fruits and vegetables that are fresh if possible. Some cities have retail stores that will deliver a box of organic food to your door once or twice a week.

- Decrease high sodium and salty foods.

- Use oil or butter instead of shortening, but use them sparingly.

- Use soy milk or rice milk instead of milk.

- Sea salt is much better to use than iodised (table) salt.

- Add nuts to increase protein content of your diet.

- Make a "snack bag" of carrot sticks, broccoli, other vegetables and nuts.

- Avoid processed or refined food as they lack nutrients.

- Do not use milk products except cream and butter in small amounts.

- Use bottled water for drinking and in cooking to avoid unhealthy micro-organisms, chlorine and fluoride.

- Cook in stainless steel and glass cookware only.

- Avoid microwave ovens, Teflon and aluminium pots and pressure cookers.

- Avoid artificial colours, flavours, preservatives, and sugar substitutes.

- Avoid alcohol, soft drinks and ice drinks (inhibits digestion).

- Avoid smoke filled rooms.

- Get a restful sleep and relaxation periods.

- Exercise daily according to your health.

- Have positive attitudes.

- Take hot baths daily to increase your circulation.

The Livingston Foundation Medical Center Meal Plan

I now do most of my shopping in a health food store or the *organic* section of a grocery store. The Livingston Foundation Medical Center recommends the following meal plan:

- Herbal teas, soy milk, rice milk

- Bread - rye, whole wheat, seven grain, corn tortillas

- Cereals - oatmeal, brown and wild rice, buckwheat.

- Dairy - heavy cream and butter in small amounts

- Desserts - fresh whole fruits, fruit cocktails, chopped apples and oranges mixed together - very good!

- Eggs: Only inoculated eggs from the Livingston Foundation Medical Center.

- Fat - olive oil, flax seed oil, fish - fresh water or deep sea fish, broiled or poached.

- Fruits - organically grown, mango, pears, grapes, apples, oranges.

- Juice - Freshly pressed only, carrot and apples and frozen pineapple juice.

Beverages

- Vegetable juices are good for the body because of the high concentration of the vegetables juiced.

- To avoid pesticides - Peel the vegetables or fruits, then scrub well with a vegetable brush; buy organic if available.

- Carrots are highly recommended, as much as one quart of juice per day. This helps build the immune system. Abscisic acid - is added to carrot juice as it helps strengthen the immune system.

- Get a good juicer. The Champion Juicer is my favorite. You receive a recipe book with the juicer so you can mix different juices. With a juicer, you can mix a combination of fruits and vegetables including carrot, cucumber, tomatoes, grapes, spinach, cabbage, beets, pineapple, cranberry, celery, strawberries, oranges, grapefruit, banana, papaya, pears, peaches, cherries, blueberries, strawberries, mangoes, onions, garlic, etc.

- I highly recommend the cookbook from the Livingston Foundation Medical Center by Anna Maria Canelas.

> **The cookbook and the Champion Juicer are also available from us.**
> **Call 1-800-665-4656**

- Meats - lamb, wild game, venison

- Nuts - unsalted, fresh, raw: Almonds, walnuts, cashews, pecans. Raw nut butter freshly made in a blender or juicer is recommended.

- Salads, raw fruits

- Sea salt, Spike, Vege-Sal

- Seasonings - fresh organic herbs or grow your own.

- Soya sauce, mustards - in moderation. Lemon juice, vegetable bouillon.

- Seeds - sunflower, sesame, flax, pumpkin - fresh and raw.

- Soup - homemade is best.

- Vegetables - organically grown, raw or fresh cooked. Especially carrots, potatoes, sweet potatoes, spinach, avocado, asparagus, peas, onion, tomatoes, lima beans, yams, swiss chard, etc.

Unhealthy Foods

- Beverages - alcohol, cocoa, coffee, soft drinks.

- Bread - White, blended bread with white flour - sprouted grain bread.

- Cereals - puffed or sugared, white rice

- Cheese - not recommended.

- Dairy - not recommended.

- Desserts - pastries, gelatines, custards, sauces, ice cream, candy, frozen fruit, canned fruit.

- Fat - shortening, margarine, saturated oils and fats.

- Fish - smoked and salted, shell fish

- Fruits - sprayed, canned or frozen

- Juices that are frozen or canned except frozen pineapple.

- Meats - chicken, beef, pork, turkey, bacon, ham and ribs. No fried, smoked, salted or processed meats, i.e. Sausages and cold cuts.

- Nuts - avoid salted; no peanuts.

- Potatoes - french-fried, and potato chips.

- Sweets - white sugar, candy, all sugar substitutes, honey.

- Vegetables - sprayed, canned, high sodium food. If fresh is not available, frozen is better than canned.

> **If your body digests higher nutrient foods, especially organic, you will feel full and satisfied with far less food**

Breakfasts

When I attended the Livingston Foundation Medical Center to build my immune system to eliminate my cancer, one of the most enjoyable experiences was eating the nutritious foods cooked by the Livingston chefs. A typical breakfast might include multi-grain whole wheat toast with very light butter, oatmeal with soy milk, or rice milk, topped with pumpkin seeds, sunflower seeds, cashews or almonds and herbal tea. For dessert, we might be served peeled apples and oranges, chopped and mixed together. The combination of the two juices tastes delicious.

> **Around 1900, one in twenty-four got cancer**
> **In the 1980's one in four got cancer**
> **In the 1990's one in three got cancer**
> **And the numbers are increasing, hence the importance of the Livingston**
> **Foundation Medical Center meal plan to build the immune system**
> **and achieve maximum health.**

Tofu cheese is also good for you. In the Livingston cookbook, there are recipes for granola, pancakes, muffins, biscuits, scrambled tofu, eggs, bread, etc. Only the Livingston eggs are recommended. However, you may use egg replacer - "non-dairy" , which comes in powdered form. Baking powder must be of the non-aluminium variety.

Sandwiches

In the Livingston cookbook, they also have a variety of sandwich recipes which I would describe as gourmet. These include vegetable sandwiches, pizza, spreads, pitas, melts, quesadilla, etc.

Salads and Dressings

The chefs at the Livingston Foundation Medical Center try to use the freshest, raw (organic) vegetables available. You can combine fresh seasonal vegetables to create salads as main course meals, or as side dishes. In the Livingston cookbook you will find recipes for potato salads, bean salads, Moroccan couscous salad, Waldorf salad, garden salad, fruit salad, and taco salad. You will find recipes for salad dressings as well, such as vinaigrettes, tofu dressing, blueberry vinaigrette, lime poppy seed, lemon, cinnamon mint, tomato herb, creamy cucumber, cashew nut, etc. You will also find recipes for salsa, mayonnaise, and guacamole.

Soups

The Livingston Foundation Medical Center stresses that canned or pre-packaged soups are abundant with artificial sweeteners, salt, meat stock, and vegetables that have lost their nutritional value. Again, ingredients for soups should be fresh and preferably organic. I buy these at my local health food store, farmer's market, or organic food section of my local grocery store. Purified drinking water should be used as there may be chemicals in tap water. The Livingston cookbook includes vegetable stock recipes so you can create your own soups. Examples of other *soup recipes* are navy bean, scallion, spinach, minestrone, zuke, miso, cream of asparagus, cauliflower, gazpacho, pea, potato, mushroom, avocado, curry red bean, Russian borscht, Moroccan lentil, cantaloupe soup, vegetable barley, carrot soup and Christmas chestnut soup. And so you can see that vegetable meal plans can be very exciting. And I am only telling you about some of the many surprises and delicious vegetarian meals in the Livingston Cookbook!

Pasta

The Livingston Foundation Medical Center suggests using one hundred percent durum pasta. Whole grain pasta with 100 % Durum as its base is best. Pasta comes in many shapes, and there is really no difference to the pasta, except the cooking time. The Livingston cookbook gives many recipes for sauces which are also good on potatoes, brown rice, and vegetables. Fresh organic vegetables are recommended with herbs and spices to enhance the flavours. A wide assortment of recipes for pasta and sauces are in the cookbook.

Vegetables

It is suggested that raw vegetables that are fresh are best for highest nourishment. If cooking, the healthiest way is to steam the vegetables until just tender. These may be served with lemon juice, pepper (white) and sea salt. The best source of organic vegetables are: your own garden, health food store, farmer's market, or organic section of your grocery store. Most recipes should combine several vegetables for highest nutrition. Never overcook vegetables. Meals based on a variety of vegetables and grains provide sufficient protein. The Livingston cookbook has 32 recipes for vegetables.

Grains and Legumes

The main source of protein on this meal plan is grains and legumes, as dairy (except a little cream and butter) are discouraged. However, you should eat legumes with grains during the same meal, as legumes are incomplete as a protein source unless complimented with a grain. When boiling dried legumes, use purified water. In the Livingston cookbook you will find many recipes such as: Greek baked beans, saffron beans, lima bean casserole, Bohemian yellow peas, tofu stew, lentils with walnuts, brown rice with mushrooms, Spanish rice, Nutted pilaff, wild rice and fresh peas, etc.

Desserts

Fresh in season fruit is the number one dessert recommended. Additional recipes are in this section, and all are made without refined sugar, white flour, or egg products. Organically grown fruit is recommended. Some recipes include tofu, arrowroot, carob powder and whole wheat flour. Nuts should be raw and unsalted. The whole fruit including peel should be used. Dried fruits must be of the unsulphured variety. Examples of dessert recipes in the Livingston cookbook include: fruit pops, fruit sorbet, frozen peach delight, strawberry banana custard, cherry pudding, apple pudding, carob pudding, sweet potato custard,

Bavarian cream with strawberries, banana split, raw fudge, carob oatmeal cookies, almond crisps, tofu cheese cake, pear pie, berry pie, apple
pie, tofu cream, whipped cream, and much more!

The Livingston Foundation Medical Center

One might describe the Livingston cookbook as an "anti-cancer diet" for
those who desire a stronger immune system. In general, you should
avoid white flour, white sugar and empty calories found in junk food
devoid of vitamins and nutrition. The foods in the cookbook are easy to
find and easy to prepare even for those who are inexperienced at cooking.

Although organic foods are more expensive, you will probably find you
will feel satisfied with smaller portions because the nutrition value of a
small portion is equal to a large portion of non-organic food. Therefore,
you can have a lot more nutrition with less food. You will likely feel psy-
chologically and physiologically full with small portions of food. Also,
the Livingston Foundation Medical Center meal plans will save you
money since they do not emphasise eating meat.

I personally love and highly recommend the Livingston lifestyle of
healthy eating. I changed my eating habits little by little, and in a short
time I found myself feeling less and less interested in foods not recommended by the Livingston Foundation Medical Center. I found that there
are many other meal plans that were a chore to follow, but this method is
easy to adopt as a lifestyle. The recipes are delicious! You will be eating
healthier foods, and you will *feel* healthier. You will benefit in your body,
mental strength and emotional control. Following the Livingston plan
with varied eating of different types of foods, you will receive all the vitamins, minerals, fats, carbohydrates, and protein that you need. What you
eat will change your life, in all areas of your life. In addition, all those illnesses related to obesity, such as heart disease, cancer, diabetes, etc. are
less likely to occur.

When I was at the Livingston Foundation Medical Center for treatment
of my cancer, I discovered that the staff themselves followed the

principles of the Livingston Foundation Medical Center, even though most have never had cancer. You do not have to follow the cookbook 100 % as that would be perfection, and that is probably asking too much of most anyone. However, if you make up your mind to follow this lifestyle of healthy *eating most of the time* you will find that your health improves more than you ever dreamed possible. There is no question that the more I follow this eating program, the healthier I feel in mind, body and control of my emotions. *Once you have changed your lifestyle of eating habits to this program you will never want to go back to the old ways of eating.*

Drink Water First, It May Be Thirst

Your body is 70% water. Without water, one will not survive more than a few days. Death can result if you lose 20 % of your body water. Water is needed for efficient movement of nutrients throughout the body, as well as for waste removal from the body. All parts of your body require lubrication to be healthy. For example, sagging skin, and wrinkles may occur after weight loss, if insufficient water is ingested during weight loss. A daily habit of drinking lots of water will make it *easier* to lose weight. Constipation is often caused by inadequate water intake.

Stress and Fluid Retention

Excessive stress can cause fluid retention. Stress may cause the release of ADH (anti-diuretic hormone), and this will result in fluid retention.

Harness Your Motivation

At first, for a day or two, make a firm decision to drink plenty of water, gradually increasing your water intake by perhaps one glass per day. Keep a diary or notepad to list how much water you drink each day. Like exercise, do not try to increase too quickly. Increase your intake of water *gradually*. Overweight folks need ten or more glasses of water daily.

Chapter 10

Why Exercise? Some Benefits:

(Read this if you ever need motivation to move your body.)

- Improve your endurance and stamina.

- Reduce your blood cholesterol.

- Improve your fitness.

- Reduce your blood pressure.

- Bring more blood and oxygen to your brain for clearer thinking.

- Reduce the risk of stroke or heart attack.

- Cope better with stress in life.

- Soothe temper.

- Have a more positive attitude.

- Make yourself happier.

- Help yourself sleep sounder, and awaken more refreshed.

- Have less fat, more muscle, and lean tissue.

- Improve digestion and function of the bowels. Important: Help clear toxins from your body so your body can more efficiently absorb nutrition from the food you eat.

- Look healthier.

- Decrease appetite - especially if you exercise one hour or more a day.

- Increase energy, vitality for life, and a feeling of well being.

- Feel healthier.

- Enjoy a stronger immune system.

- Have greater flexibility and agility.

- Have greater strength.

- Stronger bones.

- Add years to your life and life to your years.

Exercise Equipment

I use hotel gyms when travelling. However, at home, I use the equipment at my local recreation centre. It is inexpensive to attend, and you can associate with others interested in fitness and health, and you have a variety of equipment to use.

If you purchase any equipment for home use, I encourage you to buy equipment of good quality. Lesser quality equipment may lead to injury, or a breakdown of the equipment in a very short time. It is hard to lose weight. You may only burn 100 calories if you walk a mile. For example, it would take you 35 miles of walking to burn off 3500 calories, or one pound. Hard work it is, but it is well worth it!

Look at the long term picture. If you look at the low side, and lose only one pound a month, that is actually ten plus pounds a year, and fifty pounds in 5 years.

Every little bit counts, and it's better to start changing now than wishing you had done so in a year, or five years from now. Think movement! Move that body!

You can *double or triple your weight loss* by dropping the high calorie foods, such as a pat of butter at 100 calories. So, 35 pats is one less pound of fat. It all adds up! Cut those calories, especially fat calories.

Gain Weight And Lose Inches

You can actually lose inches from your waist size, yet be heavier by gaining healthy muscle. So, to increase the *speed* of your weight loss even more, do weight lifting. You can start with lesser weights and gradually increase the weights. Ask your physician about the use of weights as related to your physical condition.

A *pound* of fat is the same as a *pound* of muscle in terms of weight, but fat takes up much more space at the waist. Move that body with a varied exercise program. By using a variety of exercise, or changing your types of body movement from time to time, you will remain enthusiastic. Boredom will be impossible.

If you walked, and listened to tapes teaching a foreign language, for example, you would learn enough to be able to visit that country without an interpreter. Or, perhaps you prefer bouncy music or symphonies. Anything that increases your joy of body movement is great!

So, Be Comfortably Cool For Exercise

Too much exercise-generated heat, or excessive water loss can lead to heat stroke, brain damage, or even death. Avoid such excessive strain on your heart. Saunas and steam rooms can also be very dangerous due to the high temperatures. Any accompanying weight loss is only due to loss of water, not fat.

For warm weather, wear loose fitting, light colored clothing. For cold weather, dress in layers. Wear gloves, heavy socks and a cap to cover the head and ears.

Have Fun With Exercise

I love to walk with my walkman. It is time alone to listen to fine music, motivational tapes, comedies, and remarkable speeches. How about the fresh air, the sights, beautiful flowers, interesting people, etc?

Do what you love, and enjoy body movement. Your tastes can change too. Try new types of body movement with new choices from time to time. Your choices can stay the same, as long as you are motivated to continue your healthy body movement lifestyle.

Be Gentle On Yourself

If exercising is new to you, start with easy exercises for your physical condition, and do not go to the point of pain. A *little* pain is all right. More than that, and you are doing too much, too soon. Many people work too hard at exercise at first, and become sore or even injured, and then get too discouraged to continue their program of physical exercise. During exercise if you can't keep up a conversation with someone, you are likely exercising to a point that is currently too difficult for you.

After a while, that long walk for example, will seem shorter, and you can slowly but steadily keep increasing the activity time, speed, or intensity. Remember to stretch before and after you exercise. Never subject your body to a sudden exertion, as this could result in death. A step-by-step increase in exertion is best.

Relax Regularly

Pause several times each day. Take a long, slow, deep breath, in through your nose, and all the way down to fill up the bottom of your lungs. Then, breathe out slowly through your mouth. I always imagine I am filling up a glass at the bottom, middle and to the top. Then, I imagine emptying the glass from the top, middle, and bottom.

You can even place the palm of your hand just above your belt, and feel your body move out and in, as you breathe in and out. Those deep breaths can relax and refresh you anywhere, and even burn up a few more calories. Remember, the philosophy is that all those body movements add up to 3500 calories, and that adds up to one pound of weight loss. Keep moving, keep losing, and feel fantastic! Even if results are slow, they can be sure, and certain. Slow success is usually more permanent success. Move that body! You want to be *fit and firm forever.*

The Best Indicator

Clothes with a smaller waist that fit you will indicate your success much more than a scale. Muscle weighs more than fat. I hardly ever use a scale. The joy of slipping into clothing that I could not fit into for years is delightful.

The Best Exercise

Brisk walking is best. If you have to start slower, that's all right, but the point is to just start, and *move that body!* Just stay within the limits of your physical condition. Set a goal to gradually increase your walking speed to at least 3.5 miles per hour. This speed is good aerobic exercise and will increase your endurance. The odometer on your car can measure the distance. Gradually walk faster, or walk up hill when you wish to increase your calorie burn-up.

The Ideal Exercise Plan

1.   5 - 10 minutes warm up, and stretching.

2.   20 - 30 minutes aerobic exercise activity.

3.   5 - 10 minutes cool down, and stretching.

Follow this plan a minimum of 3 - 4 days each week. You have to exercise enough to benefit yourself, but you have to avoid exercising so hard it could damage your body. Because every person reading this book is so different in their fitness level, it would be best to discuss your involvement in selected exercises by consulting with your own physician.

Taking your pulse rate will indicate your fitness level. As you become more fit, you will notice that you maintain a slower pulse rate with the same amount of exercise.

Avoid Over-Exertion of Your Body

For example, if you do not have a warm up, and instead immediately start your session, you will cause excessive stress to the body. A heart attack could occur. Warm ups also protect against injury, and muscle soreness. So start your session with some stretching, and easy exercise to loosen your body. Similarly, do not suddenly stop your exercise, but rather slow down the pace *gradually* to make it easier on your heart.

As weeks pass, gradually add more effort to your exercise session, without excessive strain to your body. This increases your endurance level. If you miss a number of sessions due to illness, then you will have to reduce the vigour of your exercise to give your body time to return to your original level of fitness. If you stop exercising completely, you can lose all the improvement in fitness you gained, in as few as five weeks.

The Treadmill

I used to have a home gym with seven pieces of exercise equipment. My favorite was the treadmill. This is because I could read a book, watch TV, or listen to a stimulating tape on my Walkman as I walked on the treadmill. Boredom was eliminated. With a 10% incline on the treadmill, you can burn many more calories than on flat ground with the same distance and speed. If you do not hold the sidebars you will reap still greater benefits. If you need to hold on to the rails for balance, that is all right. You can gradually raise the incline on the treadmill as you become increasingly fit. Your local library likely loans lots of audiocassettes and videos for use while you exercise. Some people watch television or read.

Swimming

Walking holds first place for a best exercise. Swimming is second, as almost all muscle groups are used while swimming. It is highly beneficial for the cardio-vascular system.   Begin with 5 minutes of easy swimming for the warm up, then increase the effort expended with continuous swimming. Then, before you leave the water, slow down your pace again.

Trouble Starting Your Exercise?

Read the page titled "Why Exercise?" to motivate you. Even if you make a decision to exercise for only 5 minutes, just make a choice to "get your body moving", and you will probably want to keep exercising. The good feeling that comes from exercise acts as a reinforcer to repeat the experience.

Interval Training

If you alternate high and low exercise intensity, you will have less fatigue. For example, you could walk - jog - walk - jog, alternately every half minute or so.

Tummy Firm Up For Fast, Fabulous Results

1. Lie on your back, with your hands on your hips. Lift your legs together to a 45-degree angle, and back down, 15 times.

2. Immediately after the above, still lying flat on your back, clasp your hands behind your head. Pull your upper body up and down 15 times.

Small Meal Before Moderate Exercise

If you eat several small meals a day, and then exercise moderately, you will increase your calorie burn up. If you exercise after a *small* meal, your metabolic rate dramatically increases.

Exercise Followed By Reduced Appetite

Intense exercise usually *reduces appetite*. Your plan for a large meal may change to a desire for a small meal after vigorous exercise.

What To Take With You When You Go Walking

-   A small backpack or small handbag with some, or all of the following:

1. Water bottle - most important

2. House key

3. Money

4. Sunglasses

5. Hat

6. Sunscreen

7. Pedometer

8. Walkman cassette player

9. Tapes

10. Spare batteries

11. Kleenex or hanky

12. Pen and notepaper

Warning

Unless you are very fit, you should avoid activities that raise the heart rate too rapidly. Hence, every winter many people die shovelling snow. Such an activity may be *very* dangerous for someone who is exceedingly overweight.

Weight Plateau

You may experience quick weight loss due to water loss, then it may seem like you are not losing weight at all. Plateaus do occur often. You could worry about it, and think negative thoughts such as, "I'll never lose weight", but that will not have a positive effect on your life. It is better to affirm, "Plateaus sometimes happen. That is ok. I'll just keep working away at what I want to achieve and sooner or later, I will."

Chapter 11

Be Positive

A positive attitude is as necessary as water, food, sleep and exercise. You have to give yourself some positive thoughts everyday. If a negative thought comes into your mind, do this:

1. State the negative thought. Example: "I can't stop drinking soft drinks."

2. Disagree or affirm the opposite thought. Example: "That is ridiculous. I have stopped ... (list things you have stopped doing in the past)... before, and I can stop drinking soft drinks."

3. Substitute something more healthy. In this case, you could drink more water, carrot juice, herbal tea, etc.

4. Use future projection imagery. Imagine yourself doing whatever you should do, and as if you are the person you want to be. Like an actor, we can act *as if we* are another person. This will create new *feelings* about yourself, a new self-image. We become what we imagine with emotional intensity, clarity, and repetition.

If you ever slip back into your old ways of eating with the possibility of depression and guilt, pull up your positive attitude for weight loss and weight maintenance. Concentration is the key to all success, and we become what we focus our mental energies upon. Do your best to be optimistic, and associate with people who encourage your success. Tell yourself there are really no mistakes, but there are *learning experiences*.

Believe in yourself, and your hidden, untapped strengths which are about to be released. Realise that you have learned much in all those years of living that will help you to sustain your motivation to attain the success you desire. Norman Vincent Peale said: "Walk with your head held high and be victorious."

When you *think* positive, you begin to *feel* positive. This is because you release different chemicals in your body by your different thoughts. So, we are largely the boss, writer, and director of our feelings. Control your thoughts to control your feelings, and you will control your actions and behaviour.

Positive Affirmations

You can *decide* to think more positively in your *daily life*. You can also affirm positive thoughts in *self-hypnosis*. Affirmations should be positive, stating only what you want to do, and not what you do not want to do. Examples:

- "I am becoming more slim everyday."

- "I am satisfied with small, reasonable portions of food."

- "It's easy for me to stick to my program."

- "I find it easy to keep my new lifestyle habits, and I will remain trim permanently."

- "I chew my food slowly, thoroughly, completely."

Note: One physician told me he recommends chewing each bite of food *50 times!* This results in less work for your digestive system. You will be healthier and feel full with less food. This is fantastic advice. However, I personally found it difficult to keep food in my mouth that long without my body automatically wanting to swallow. The point is to chew your food as much as possible, to improve your digestion, and to feel full with less food.

Chapter 12

When Life Is Not Fair

Life is often not fair. Dr. Milton Erickson tells the story of when he was a young medical student, and he had to face the fact that life is not fair. He was thinking about how some people are healthy, and really do nothing positive in their life. Yet, here in his office was a beautiful, kind, young girl who he knew had a disease that would soon take her life.

You may have catastrophes in your life such as family problems, health problems, financial problems, and other personal difficulties. This does make life unfair, and tough to face. All you can do is follow the advice I've given when I discussed handling stress. My favourites are talking to others, especially a good counsellor, self-help tapes, deep breathing, exercise, progressive relaxation by tensing and relaxing individual muscles, and massage. Sometimes I go into self-hypnosis, and ask my creative subconscious to answer questions or to provide solutions for me. I might simply ask my subconscious "What should I do to solve this challenge?" Although difficulties and challenges occur in everyone's life, we have to ask ourselves how we should view the difficulty and what is best to lessen the consequences of it. We always have some choices left.

I personally know unfairness, and a tough life. In 1996, within a few short months, I simultaneously experienced divorce papers, harassment by lawyers, mountains of legal papers that made me a single father, the loss of over half of my 40 years of savings, the return of a knee problem that forced me to walk with a cane, rapid heartbeat, failing eyesight, rapid weight loss, diagnosis that I had a hyperthyroid condition, and then thyroid cancer.

So, you see what excessive stress can do. Fortunately, my children are healthy, and my cancer has disappeared. However, I continue, for life to take a daily thyroid pill, and inject myself with immune building "potions", and am fairly careful about what I eat, breathe, drink, and place upon my skin. However, if you compare your difficulties with those of others in countries ravaged by war, earthquakes, disease, and starvation, our challenges grow smaller.

The Passage Of Time Is Also A Strong Healer

What mattered five or ten years ago is of little thought today. The most important part is you. If you can say "I am still here, alive and able to enjoy the wonders that surround me", how wonderful!

Thyroid Pills

Many people take thyroid pills for hypothyroidism. When my thyroid gland was removed, I became hypothyroid for life and dependant upon this daily pill. At first I found it very difficult to keep the weight off. As my doctor constantly checked my TSH reading in my blood every few months, he would prescribe a new thyroid medication. Finally, the right level was determined for me, and I found it to be possible to control my weight, but it is still not easy. I do have to be careful what I eat, and to move my body! It is possible that you may come out of life's catastrophes stronger than ever! I learned a lot from those tough years when life was not fair.

Dropping Worries

If you have concerns that harass you, see a *good* professional who specialises in solving problems in your area of concern. If you have friends or relatives asking for your help, and you cannot help, stop worrying. Tell them to see such a specialist in their area of concern. Taking too many of the world's problems on our shoulders can kill us by excessive stress. Ask yourself: "What does it cost me to think negative thoughts? What rewards will I get when I think in a positive way, about the present and the future? What goals can I set for myself? What *plans* can I make to reach those goals? What can I *do* to make those plans successful?"

My Positive Attitudes Are:

(Fill in with an erasable pencil, or photocopy this page so you can revise your affirmations from time to time):

_____

_____

_____

_____

_____

_____

_____

_____

_____

_____

_____

Instead of saying to yourself, "I wish ….. or if only ….., then things would be alright", *take control of your life*. Accept responsibility for your future and say, "What can I do now?" Or better yet, "How can I improve my life because of this?" **You may not be able to control yesterday, but you can control this present moment.**

What if Life's Stresses and Emotional Challenges Are Absolutely Unmanageable?

Please see your physician right away. Sometimes meditation, hypnosis, massage, deep breathing, etc., are not enough. Your physician may prescribe medication for temporary use, and refer you to a good therapist.

"Because one never

knows how long one

has on the beautiful

and most fascinating

planet earth,

I always say,

enjoy every moment"

From *The Wellness Journey*

By M. Vance Romane

Chapter 13

Making Success As Certain As The Sun Rises Each Day!

What If...Blah, Blah, Blah

I've been giving seminars for over 35 years, and here's what keeps people from attending, or doing what they need to do for success. They will use their dynamic mind power imagination in a negative way, and say to themselves, "What if it does not work?", "What if I gain all the weight back again", "How will I change my family's habits?", and on, and on. If this negative self-talk energy and imagination was used to *get started on a planned action*, success would be given a chance to happen.

Your Energy Level

With proper nutrients, exercise and no interfering illnesses, there is no reason to feel tired. If you do, then you must consult with your physician. And think positive too. To create energy for the coming day, I often lie in bed at night, and before sleep, I imagine that I am going through the next day's routine activities feeling strong, energetic, full of enthusiasm, positive thoughts, and a joy for living.

A Merry And Joyful Heart

Happiness adds to health. What makes one person happy may not be enough for another person. If you ever feel sorry for yourself because you lack something, focus upon what you do have. Focus upon how lucky you really are living in a relatively prosperous, and safe country.

Increase your joy for life with regular PHYSICAL exercise; MENTAL or INTELLECTUAL pursuits; a POSITIVE OUTLOOK on life; and enjoyment of the SIGHTS, SOUNDS, SCENTS, TASTES, and FEELINGS that are abundant everywhere for your experience. Friends and intimate relationships add to the joy of living. When you are happier, it is easier to make healthy choices and to affirm success. I just do my best to make each day a little bit better for myself and others.

New Interests

I am never bored. I always have something to do. A lot of interests will move thoughts away from eating. Again, consider your maxim to be **"I eat to live, but I do not live to eat."** With a sense of curiosity about the wonders of our world, you can seek new experiences, and pursue so many interests unrelated to food, to replace the unhealthy with the healthy. Often experiences you never thought you would enjoy can become a regular pastime. Try it! You might like it! So develop lots of interests other than food.

> I **_WILL_** DO IT!

Persistence For Success

You can be a talented, educated genius, but that alone will not give you a firm, fit body forever. Only the will to succeed, determination, and persistence will make your endeavour successful. Believe in yourself! **Do it!**

> **You can't control your past – but you can control your future**

DO IT FOR YOU!

Wishing you a long life filled to the brim with
health, happiness and prosperity!
Your friend,
M. Vance Romane

Bibliography and References

Adams, Paul. *The New Self-Hypnosis.* Hollywood: Wilshire Book Company, 1975.

Alman, Vance M., and Lambrou, Peter. *Self-Hypnosis: The Complete Manual For Health and Self-Change.* New York: Brunner/Mazel, Publishers, 1992.

Araoz, Daniel L. *The New Hypnosis.* New York: Brunner/Mazel Inc., 1985.

Arluck, Edward Wiltcher. *Hypnoanalysis: a Case Study.* New York: Random House, 1964.

Arons, Harry. *Handbook of Self-Hypnosis.* Irvington: Power Publishers, 1969.

Bailey, Covert, and Bishop, Lea, *The Fit Or Fat Woman,* Boston: Houghton Mifflin, 1989.

Bailey, Covert, *How to Get Fit Fast,* Video, Los Angeles: Pacific Arts, 1993.

Bailey, Covert, *Living Smart Staying Healthy,* Niles: Nightingale-Conant Corp., 1996.

Bandler, Richard and Grinder, John. *Patterns of the Hypnotic Techniques of Milton H. Erickson, M.D.,* Cupertino: Meta Publications, 1975.

Barabasz, Dr. Arreed F. *New Techniques in Behavior Therapy and Hypnosis.* South Orange: Power Publishers, Inc., 1977.

Barnard, Neal, *Foods That Cause You To Lose Weight,* Texas: The Magni Group, 1992.

Beaulieu, Michael S., *Obesity, A Disease of the Mind,* New Haven: Prometheus Bound, 1986.

Bowers, Kenneth S. *Hypnosis for the Seriously Curious,* New York/London: W.W. Norton & Company, 1976.

Boyne, Gil. *How to Teach Self-Hypnosis.* Robert S. Fraser, Editor, 1987.

Boyne, Gil. *Hypnosis: New Tool in Nursing Practice.* Glendale: Westwood Publishing Company, 1982.

Bricklin, Mark, and Gerus, Claire, *Lose Weight Guidebook,* Emmaus: Rodale Press, Inc., 1994.

Bricklin, Mark, *Lose Weight Naturally,* Emmaus: Rodale Press, Inc., 1989.

Bristol, Claude M. *The Magic of Believing.* New York: Pocket Books, 1972.

Brooks, C.H. *Self Mastery Through Conscious Auto Suggestion by Emile Coue & the Practice of Autosuggestion by the Method of Emile Coue.* London: George Allen & Unwin, 1984.

Caprio, Frank S., and Berger, Joseph R. *Helping yourself with Self-Hypnosis.* New York: Warner Paperback Library, 1975.

Cheek, David B., M.D., and LeCron, Leslie M. *Clinical Hypnotherapy*. New York: Grune & Stratton, Inc., 1968.

Chertok, L. *Hypnosis*. Toronto: Pergamon Press, 1966.

Citrenbaum, Charles M. *Weight Control Through Trance and Self-hypnosis*. New York: W. W. Norton and Company, 1985.

Citrenbaum, Charles M., King, Mark E., and William, I. Cohen, *Modern Clinical Hypnosis for Habit Control*, New York: W.W. Norton and Company, 1985.

Clarke, Christopher and Jackson, J. Arthur. *Hypnosis and Behavior Therapy*. New York: Springer Publishing Company, Inc., 1983.

Cooke, C.E. and Van Vogt, A.E. *Hypnotism Handbook*. Alhambra: Borden Publishing Co., 1965.

Cott, Allan, M.D., Fasting: *The Ultimate Diet*, New York: Bantam Books, 1975.

Coue, Emile. *How to Practice Suggestion and Autosuggestion*. New York: American Library Service, 1923.

Crasilneck, H.B., and Hall, J.A. *Clinical Hypnosis Principal and Applications*. New York: Grune and Stratton, 1975.

Crook, Marion, *The Body Image Trap*, Vancouver: Self-Counsel Press, 1991.

Debetz, Barbara, M.D. *Your Diet Coach*. New York: Prentice Hall Press, 1989.

DeVore, Steven A., *The Neuropsycholoy of Weight Control* (audio cassette album), Newark: Syber Visions Systems, 1985.

Dorcus, Roy M. *Hypnosis and Its Therapeutic Applications*. Toronto: McGraw-Hill Book Company, Inc., 1956.

Dowd, E. Thomas and Healy, James M. *Case Studies in Hypnotherapy*. New York: The Guilford Press, 1986.

Duckworth, John. *How to Use Auto-Suggestion Effectively*. Hollywood: Wilshire Book Company, 1976.

Edmunds, Simeon. *The Psychic Power of Hypnosis*. London: The Aquarian Publishing Co. Ltd., 1978.

Eisenberg, Howard. *Inner Spaces*. Parapsychological Explorations of the Mind. Don Mills: Musson Book Company, 1977.

Ellen, Arthur. *The Intimate Casebook of a Hypnotist*. Toronto: The New American Library of Canada Limited, 1968.

Ellis, Albert, Abrams, Michael, and Dengelegi, Lidia, *The Art and Science of Rational Eating*, Fort Lee: Barricade Books Inc., 1992.

Elman, Dave. *Hypnotherapy*. Los Angeles: Westwood Publishing Co., 1964.

Erickson, Milton H. Experiencing *Hypnosis - Therapeutic Approaches to Altered States*. New York: Irvington Publishers, Inc., 1981.

Erickson, Milton H. *Hypnotic Realities*. New York: Irvington Publishers, Inc., 1976.

Erickson, Milton H. *Innovative Hypnotherapy*. Volumes 1,2,3&4. New York: Irving Publishers, Inc., 1980.

Erickson, Milton H. *My Voice Will Go With You*. New York: Norton & Company, 1982.

Erickson, Milton H.; Hershman, Seymour; and Secter, Irving I. *Medical And Dental Hypnosis*. New York: The Julian Press, Inc., 1961.

Evans, Elizabeth, *Diet and Nutrition*, New York: Exeter Books, 1979.

Gendlin, Eugene T. *Focusing*. Toronto: Bantam Books, Inc., 1981.

Gibson, Walter. *Hypnotism Theory and Practice*. Toronto: Coles Publishing Company, 1979.

Gibson, Walter. *Hypnotism Through The Ages.* New York: Vista House Publishers, 1961.

Gibson, Walter. *The Key to Hypnotism.* Baltimore: Ottenheimer Publishers, Inc., 1956.

Grouch, David A., M.D., and Fross, Garland H. *What Every Subject Should Know About Hypnosis and Self-Hypnosis.* South Orange: Power Publishers, Inc., 1976.

Gutwirth, Samuel W. *You Can Learn to Relax.* North Hollywood: Wilshire Book Company, 1974.

Hadley, Josie and Staudacher, Carol. *Hypnosis for Change.* New York: Ballantine Books, 1987.

Haley, Jay. *Uncommon Therapy*. New York: W.W. Norton & Company, 1973.

Hansen, Carol, *Lighten Up Inspirations*, Concord: Open Heart Press, 1998

Hart, Hornell. *Autoconditioning: The New Way to a Successful Life.* Englewood Cliffs: Prentice Hall, Inc., 1977.

Heidrich, Ruth, *A Race For Life*, Honolulu: Heidrich Weisbrod Association, 1990

Heidrich, Ruth, *The Race For Life Cookbook*, Honolulu: Hawaii Health Pubishers, 1994.

Heise, Jack, *The Amazing Hypno Diet*, New York: Belmont Books, 1962.

Heron William T., and Hershman, Seymour. *An Old Art Returns to Medicine.* 1958.

Hirsh, Alan R. M.D., *Dr. Hirsch's Guide To Scentsational Weight Loss*, Dorset: Element Books Limited, 1997.

Hoke, James H. *I Would If I Could And I Can. Program Your Personality for Success.* New York: Berkley Books, 1982.

Hollander, Bernard, M.D. *Methods and Uses of Hypnosis and Self-Hypnosis.* Hollywood: Wilshire Book Company, 1978.

Hunt, Douglas, *No More Cravings*, New York: Warner Books, 1987.

Hypnovision, *Weight Loss Video*, Boston: Self Improvement Video Inc., 1984.

Johnson, Debbie, *Think Yourself Thin*, New York: Harper Collins Publishers, 1996.

Jourard, Sidney M. *The Transparent Self*. Toronto: D. Van Nostrand Company (Canada) Ltd., 1964.

Kappas, John G. *Professional Hypnotism Manual*. Panorama City: Panorama Publishing Company, 1978.

Kirtley, Christine. *Consumer Guide to Hypnosis*. Merrimack: The National Guild of Hypnotists, 1991.

Kline, Milton V. *Freud and Hypnosis The Interaction of Psychodymanics and Hypnosis*. New York: The Julian Press, Inc., 1958.

Klippstein, Hildegard. *Ericksonian Hypnotherapeutic Group Inductions*. New York: Brunner/Mazel Publishers, 1991.

Koop, C. Everett, *Overweight and Obesity*, Video, New York: Time Life Medical, 1996.

Kraus, Barbara, *Calories and Carbohydrates*, New York: New American Library, Inc., 1975.

Kroger, William S., M.D. *Clinical and Experimental Hypnosis*. Toronto: J.B. Lippincott Company, 1977.

Kroger, William S., M.D. *Hypnosis and Behavior Modification: Imagery Conditioning*. Toronto: J.B. Lippincott Company, 1976.

Kuntzleman and Runyon, *The Perfect Way To Lose Weight*, Wheaton: Tyndale House Publishers, Inc., 1986.

Lankton, Stephen R. and Carol H. *The Answer Within: A Clinical Framework of Ericksonian Hypnotherapy*. New York: Brunner/Mazel, Publishers, 1983.

LeCron, Leslie M. *Self Hypnotism The Technique and Its Use in Daily Living*. New York: The New American Library, 1964.

LeCron, Leslie M. *Techniques of Hypnotherapy*. New York: The Julian Press, 1961.

LeCron, Leslie M. *The Complete Guide to Hypnosis*. New York: Barnes and Noble Books, 1973.

Lindner, Peter, M.D., *Mind Over Platter*, Beverly Hills: Hal Leighton Printing Co., 1963.

Lindner, Peter, M.D., and Daisy, *Dr. Lindner's Point System Food Program*, Hollywood: Wilshire Book Company, 1976.

Macrae, Janet. *Therapeutic Touch, A Practical Guide*. New York: Alfred A. Knopf, 1988.

Magonet, Phillip, M.D. *Practical Hypnotism*. Hollywood: Wilshire Book Company, 1976.

Marcuse, F.L. *Hypnosis Fact and Fiction*. Baltimore: Penguin Books Ltd., 1971.

Morris, Freda. *Self-Hypnosis in Two Days*. New York: E.P. Dutton & Co., Inc., 1975.

Moss, C. Scott. *Hypnosis in Perspective*. Toronto: Collier-Macmillan, 1965.

Mutke, Peter H.C., M.D. *Selective Awareness*. Millbrae: Celestial Arts, 1977.

Napowsa, Walters D. *Hypno-Technology: Roles of the Hypno-Technician*. St. Petersburg: S.O.S. Printing, 1977.

New Haven Hypnotherapy, *Hypnotherapy in Bariatrics*, New Haven Hypnotherapy, 1990.

Nightingale, Earl. *The New Lead The Field*. (audiocassette album) Chicago: Nightingale-Conant Corporation.

Oechsli, Matt, *Autohypnosis "Diet"*, New York, Sterling Publishing Company, 1990.

Older, Jules *Touching is Healing*. New York: Stein and Day/Publishers, 1982.

Orton, Louis J. *Hypnotism Made Practical*. Hollywood: Wilshire Book Company, 1976.

Parker, Jonathan, *Winning At Losing*, Ojai, Ca.: Gateways Research Institute, 1986.

Peale, Norman Vincent and Robert Clifford. *Live Longer And Better*. Foundation for Christian Living.

Petrie, Sidney. *What Modern Hypnotism Can Do For You*. Greenwich: Fawcett Publications, Inc., 1972.

Petrie, Sidney and Stone, Robert B. *How To Reduce and Control Your Weight Through Self-hypnotism*, Englewood Cliffs: Parker Publishing Company, Inc., 1965.

Petrie, Sidney and Stone, Robert B. *Hypno Cybernetics*. Helping Yourself to a Rich New Life. Englewood Cliffs: Parker Publishing Company, Inc., 1976.

Powers, Melvin. *Advanced Techniques of Hypnosis*. Hollywood: Wilshire Book Company, 1978.

Powers, Melvin. *Hypnotism Revealed*. Hollywood: Wilshire Book Company, 1978.

Powers, Melvin and Starrett, Robert S. *A Practical Guide to Better Concentration*. Hollywood: Wilshire Book Company, 1962.

Powter, Susan, Eating, *Information to Get You Started*, Susan Powter Corp., 1993.

Powter, Susan, *Give Me A Minute*, Dallas: Susan Powter Corp., 1992.

Powter, Susan, *Stop The Insanity*, Dallas: Susan Powter Corp., 1992.

Pritikin, Nathan, *Diet For Runners*, New York: Simon and Schuster, 1982.

Prudden, Suzy, *Change Your Mind, Change Your Body*, New York: Harper Collins Publishers, 1992.

Prudden, Suzy. *Meta Fitness: Your Thoughts Taking Shape.* Santa Monica: Hay House Inc., 1989.

Pulos, Lee. *Beyond Hypnosis.* Vancouver: Omega Press, 1990.

Ray, Sondra, *The Only Diet There Is,* Berkeley: George Banta Company, 1981.

Reardon, William T., M.D. *Modern Medical Hypnosis.* Wilmington, 1965.

Rodale Press, *The Good Fats,* Emmaus: Rodale Press, 1989.

Rubin, Isaac, M.D., *The Thin Book,* New York: Pinnacle Books, 1966.

Ruby, Glenda, *The Beverly Hillbillies Diet,* New York, Beaufort Books, Inc., 1982

Schneck, Jerome M. *Hypnosis In Modern Medicine.* Springfield: Charles C. Thomas, 1963.

Schwartz, Bob, *Diets Don't Work,* Las Vegas: Breakthru Publishing, 1986.

Segall, Martin M. *The Questions They Ask.* South Orange: Power Publishers, Inc., 1975.

Shames, Richard, M.D. and Sterin, Chuck. *Healing With Mind Power.* Emmaus: Rodale Press, 1978.

Silva, Jose. *The Silva Mind Control Method.* New York: Pocket Books, 1978.

Simonson, Maria, and Heilman, Joan Rattner, *The Complete University Medical Diet,* New York: Rawson Associates, 1983.

Simonton, O. Carl M.D. *Getting Well Again.* Los Angeles: J.P. Tarcher, Inc., 1978.

Straus, Roger A. *Creative Self-Hypnosis.* New York/London: Prentice Hall Press, 1989.

Sutphen, Dick, *Holophonic Weight Loss Audio Cassettes,* Malibu: Valley of the Sun, 1989.

Tebbetts, Charles. *Self-Hypnosis and Other Mind Expanding Techniques.* Glendale: Westwood Publishing Company, 1977.

Tebbetts, Charles. *Miracles on Demand.* The Radical Short-Term Hypnotherapy of Gil Boyne. Glendale: Westwood Publishing Company, 1987.

Tracy, David *How to Use Hypnosis.* New York: Sterling Publishing Company, 1952.

Tyson, Mary Catherine, M.D., and Robert, *The Psychology Of Successful Weight Control,* Chicago: Nelson-Hall Company, 1974.

Ulene, Art, *Keep It Off Today,* National Broading Company, 1995.

Van Pelt, S.J., M.D. *Secrets of Hypnotism.* Hollywood: Wilshire Book Company, 1976.

Vartabedian, Roy E. and Matthews, Kathy. *Nutripoints, The Breakthrough Point System for Optimal Nutrition.* New York: Harper and Row Publishers, 1982.

Wilson, Donald L., M.D. *Total Mind Power*. Los Angeles: Camero Publishing Co 1976.

Weil, Andres, *8 Weeks To Optimum Health*, Seattle: Inner Dimension, 1997.

Weitzenhoffer, Andre. *Modern Hypnosis*. Hollywood: Wilshire Book Company, 1977.

Whitlock, Jennifer, Editor, *Lose Weight Naturally Newsletter, Emmaus*, PA., Lose Weight Naturally, 1989

Wynn, Ralph. *Hypnotism Made Easy*. Hollywood: Wilshire Book Company, 1978.

Young, L.E. *25 Lessons in Hypnotism*. New York: Padell Book Company, 1963.

Zeig, Jeffrey K. *Ericksonian Approaches to Hypnosis and Psychotherapy*. New York: Brunner/Mazel, Publishers, 1982.

Zilbergeld, Bernie and Lazarus, Arnold A. *Mind Power: Getting What You Want Through Mental Training*. Toronto: Little, Brown and Company, 1987.

Romane Self-Help, Home-Use Programs

Romane Hypnosis Cassettes:

Only $15.00 each. *Warning: Do not play any Hypnosis Audio Cassette Recordings while driving.*

1. Enjoy Dental Visits With No Fear, No Pain / I Believe in Myself.

2. Positive Mental Attitude / Confidence at Job Interviews. For those seeking employment.

3. Better Memory / Be Motivated To Study.

4. Enjoy Exercise / Enjoy Good Health.

5. Have Fun Experiencing Past Lives / Astral Energising - A Trip Without The Ticket.

6. End Procrastination / Overcome Fear Of Failure.

7. Develop Powerful Concentration / Be Relaxed During Examinations.

8. Cut Down Or Stop Drinking Alcohol / For Men: End Sexual Impotence.

9. Better Golfing / Better Bowling.

10. Fall Asleep Easily / Banish Worry.

11. Enjoy Housework / Use The Power Of Colours To Change Your Life.

12. Be a Great Conversationalist / Make Friends Easily.

13. Stop Nail Biting / Be More Assertive and Confident.

14. Increase Energy and Enthusiasm / Best of Health.

15. Forget Negative Images Of The Past / Achieve Maximum Happiness.

16. Money Magnet Mind For Prosperity / Program Your Mind For Success.

17. For Women: Love Your Body / Enhance Self-Esteem.

18. Secrets of Creativity / Be a Successful Problem Solver.

19. Stop Stuttering and Speak Confidently / Be a Dynamic Public Speaker.

20. Develop Better Imagery / Faster Success.

21. Banish Jealousy / Be Forgiving To Yourself And Others.

22. Reach Your Goals / Develop Enthusiasm.

23. Eliminate Tension Headaches With Several Mind Power Methods.

24. Perfection in Piano. Play Your Best and Be Relaxed During Exams, Recitals and Performances.

MUSIC FOR RELAXATION, MEDITATION, MASSAGE & PEACE OF MIND

25. Side A: Astral Violet by Sondra Gordon. Side B: Past, Present, Future by Christoper Lee Pavlik.

26. Side A: Ocean Sounds by Tony Scrace. Side B: Journey Within by Tony Scrace.

VIDEO TAPE SETS:

Complete Stop Smoking Seminar - Three Videos - $125.00

- TAPE ONE: Fact and Fiction About Hypnosis, Creating the Hypnotic Mood. TAPE TWO: Mind Power Training, Hypnotic Conditioning, Bonus! Stress Control and Self-Esteem Building. TAPE THREE: Virtually The World's Most Powerful Hypnosis Session To Stop Smoking.

Complete Lose Weight Seminar - Three Videos - $125.00

- TAPE ONE: Fact and Fiction About Hypnosis, Creating the Hypnotic Mood

  TAPE TWO: Mind Power Training, Hypnotic Conditioning, Bonus! Stress Control and Self-Esteem Building. TAPE THREE: Virtually The World's Most Powerful Hypnosis Session To Lose Weight.

AUDIO CASSETTE TAPE SETS:

Complete Stop Smoking Seminar - Four Cassettes OR CD's - $80.00

- 3 Cassettes running about 2 hours, with a complete seminar recorded live and an additional 4th tape for reinforcement to keep you a permanent non-smoker.

Complete Lose Weight Seminar - Three Cassettes - $60.00

- 2 Cassettes running about 2 hours, with a complete seminar recorded live. Plus an additional tape for reinforcement and weight maintenance.

Self-Hypnosis Seminar - Three Cassettes - $60.00

- Learn about hypnosis and why it works. Master self-hypnosis by being hypnotized with post-hypnotic suggestion. Learn how to give yourself hypnotic suggestions to overcome unhealthy habits and to achieve your maximum personal best. 2 cassettes, and printed material, plus a third cassette, the Energy Refresher. About 3 hours.

Stress Control Workshop - Four Cassettes - $80.00

- 3 Cassettes of a seminar running over 2 hours. Life has constant invitations to stress, the unseen killer. Enjoy greater peace of mind, be calm and be relaxed with over 20 methods. Overcome needless worry, sleep better, enjoy the best of health in mind and body. Includes a 4th cassette, a "reinforcer".

Books:

The Wellness Journey Book, By M. Vance Romane - $15.00

- Through hypnosis, Romane shows people how to reach their inner strength to overcome problems and actualise their dreams with the power of self-hypnosis.

To Order:

Please list titles desired adding $3.50 shipping for the first item and $.50 for each additional item. Please also add applicable sales taxes. To order or to contact Romane for a speaking engagement, seminars, or special presentations write:

M. Vance Romane c/o M.V.P. Ltd.

In Canada: In USA:

PO Box 75177   PMB 268
White Rock Postal Outlet   250 H. St.
White Rock, BC   Blaine, Wa.
V4B 5L4   98230

Phone: 1-800-665-4656

Fax: 604-538-8477

Web Page: www.vanceromane.com

PS. You are invited to write to Romane if you have any questions.